# Safety Testing of New Drugs

# Safety Testing of New Drugs

## Laboratory predictions and clinical performance

*Edited by*

### D. R. LAURENCE, MD, FRCP
*Professor of Pharmacology & Therapeutics,*
*School of Medicine,*
*University College, London, U.K.*

### A. E. M. McLEAN, BM, PhD, FRCPath.
*Professor of Toxicology,*
*School of Medicine,*
*University College, London, U.K.*

### M. WEATHERALL, DM, DSc, FIBiol.
*formerly Head of Therapeutic Research Division,*
*Director of Establishment,*
*Wellcome Research Laboratories, Beckenham, U.K.*

1984

ACADEMIC PRESS
*Harcourt Brace Jovanovich, Publishers*
London   Orlando
San Diego   San Francisco   New York   São Paulo
Sydney   Tokyo   Toronto   Montreal

ACADEMIC PRESS INC. (LONDON) LTD.
24/28 Oval Road
London NW1

*United States Edition published by*
ACADEMIC PRESS INC.
(Harcourt Brace Jovanovich, Inc.)
Orlando, Florida 32887

**British Library Cataloguing in Publication Data**

Safety testing of new drugs.
  1. Drugs—Safety measures 2. Drugs
  —Testing
  I. Laurence, D. R.   II. McLean, A. E. M.
  III. Weatherall, M.
  363.1′9464    RS189

  ISBN 0-12-438350-5

  LCCN 83-83426

Typeset by Paston Press, Norwich
Printed in Great Britain by
St Edmundsbury Press, Bury St Edmunds, Suffolk

# Contributors

H. K. Adam, *ICI PLC, Pharmaceuticals Division, Alderley Park, Macclesfield, Cheshire SK10 3DT, England.*

R. W. Brimblecombe, *Smith, Kline and French Research Limited, The Frythe, Welwyn, Herts AL6 9AR, England.*

J. M. Cruikshank, *ICI PLC, Pharmaceutical Division, Alderley Park, Macclesfield, Cheshire SK10 3DT, England.*

J. D. Fitzgerald, *ICI PLC, Pharmaceutical Division, Alderley Park, Macclesfield, Cheshire SK10 3DT, England.*

E. Flückiger, *Preclinical Research Department, Pharmaceutical Division, Sandoz Limited, CH-4002 Basel, Switzerland.*

A. F. Green, *Wellcome Research Laboratories, Langley Court, Beckenham, Kent BR3 3BS, England.*

D. R. Laurence, *Department of Clinical Pharmacology, The Rayne Institute, 5 University Street, London WC1E 6JJ, England.*

G. B. Leslie, *Smith, Kline and French Research Limited, The Frythe, Welwyn, Herts AL6 9AR,* England.

A. E. M. McLean, *Department of Clinical Pharmacology, The Rayne Institute, 5 University Street, London WC1E 6JJ, England.*

J. S. Patterson, *ICI PLC, Pharmaceuticals Division, Alderley Park, Macclesfield, Cheshire SK10 3DT, England.*

B. P. Richardson, *Preclinical Research Department, Pharmaceutical Division, Sandoz Limited, CH-4002 Basel, Switzerland.*

M. J. Tucker, *ICI PLC, Pharmaceutical Division, Alderley Park, Macclesfield, Cheshire SK10 3DT, England.*

I. Turkalj, *Drug Monitoring Centre, Pharmaceutical Division, Sandoz Limited, CH-4002 Basel, Switzerland.*

M. Weatherall, *Wellcome Research Laboratories, Langley Court, Beckenham, Kent BR3 3BS, England.*

# Contents

# 1

# Introduction

D. R. LAURENCE, A. E. M. McLEAN and M. WEATHERALL

When a doctor prescribes a drug, he should be aware of the specific effects he hopes to achieve and of the unwanted effects which will occur if the dose is too high or the patient reacts abnormally. He will probably take for granted that the drug will not cause any of a very large number of possible unwanted effects in the individual before him, and he will nearly always be right in this respect. However, in the last fifty years, many new drugs have been introduced. Among them a few have caused grave alarm by producing serious unwanted and unexpected effects. Some of these have remained in use, but others have been withdrawn with losses to therapeutics and to their manufacturers. An enormous amount of labour has been expended on devising tests *in vitro* and experiments on living animals to make quite sure that there will be no more serious alarms or accidents. But the results of this labour have been sadly disappointing. The number of valuable new drugs introduced has declined (May *et al.* 1983), but the proportion which have caused alarm has probably changed very little. However, the procedures intended to confer greater safety have become enshrined in the legal requirements of many countries, although their efficacy is questionable. The purpose of this work is to examine the procedures which were adopted for a number of undoubtedly useful new drugs marketed more than seven years ago, and to see how far subsequent experience in the clinical use of the drugs has reflected benefits from the testing procedures adopted.

New drugs are valuable for the cure or alleviation of previously incurable diseases, and as part of the stepwise improvement of existing remedies of all kinds. The discovery of new drugs can happen in various ways, ranging from chance observation to planned research. But the full development and manufacture of potential new remedies needs resources which only the pharmaceutical industry provides. In the course of its activities in the last century or so, the industry has had many successes and some disasters, of which the thalidomide tragedy is the most notable. The disasters have led to increasing attempts by the industry to detect potential dangers of new remedies before they are made widely available (Report, 1964) and to very substantial growth of government regulations in most of the developed nations of the world (Report, 1966). The regulations are now seen in many quarters to have become excessive, to the extent of hampering the introduction of valuable drugs without conferring the hoped-for benefits of greater safety (Report, 1976; Lasagna, 1979; Weatherall, 1982).

Among the reasons for this situation is the lack of standing of toxicology as an experimental science relevant to man. It is obviously dangerous and impractical to administer new chemical entities to humans with no knowledge of their pharmacological and toxicological properties, and the necessary information is obtained by experiments in animals. Such information is, broadly considered, of great value, but variations in the reactions of different species, and of individuals within a species limit the predictive reliability of such evidence. Many toxicologists work entirely in laboratories remote from the practice of medicine and do not have experience of real clinical problems. Extrapolation from data obtained in animals is liable to be naive in such conditions. As long as favourable properties are being studied, the worst that can go wrong is that a substance, promising in animals, does not work so well in man, and little is lost by its trial. But if a substance has unfavourable properties in animals, there is a *prima facie* incentive to caution which may lead to abandonment of a good remedy before its benefits are properly assessed and its risks understood.

The methods of assessing toxicity in animals are largely empirical and unvalidated (Report, 1978). It has become common practice to use large numbers of animals in each experiment, so they are costly. Most of the experiments are done in industrial laboratories and the information obtained has considerable commercial value; it is submitted in confidence to regulatory authorities, and much of it is usually not made public. For both these reasons, the ordinary criterion of scientific reliability (that the results are reproducible in other laboratories) does not operate. The details are not widely known, and the cost of further experiments on the same lines is prohibitive even if there are good academic or commercial reasons for doing them. When the methodology of conventional test procedures is discussed it becomes evident that quite small differences in procedure can have large effects on the outcome, and so on the inferences which may be drawn from them. It is urgently necessary to know whether the tests as in fact conducted have sufficient predictive value to be justifiable, or whether they are a colossal waste of resources to no good purpose.

In order to make such judgements, a number of case histories have been assembled with details of the experiments done in animals, the predictions made from them before the substance tested was administered to man, and the actual outcome both in terms of therapeutic benefit and of ill-effects whether predicted or unforeseen. These case histories have been provided by the courtesy of four pharmaceutical companies—Imperial Chemical Industries plc, Sandoz Ltd, Smith, Kline and French Laboratories Ltd. and the Wellcome Foundation Ltd. Their publication is a substantial departure from normal practice, and we are deeply grateful to the companies for their generous collaboration. This sequence of reports, and possibly more to follow, will provide a source of "case-law", invaluable in planning future studies and in deciding whether any particular procedure has, in fact, ever conferred some worthwhile protection which justified its cost.

# References

Lasagna, L. (1979). Toxicological barriers to providing better drugs. *Arch. Toxicol.* **43**, 27–33.

May, M. S., Wardell, W. M. and Lasagna, L. (1983). New drug development during and after a period of regulatory change: Clinical research activity of major United States pharmaceutical firms, 1958 to 1979. *Clin. Pharmacol. Ther.* **33**, 691–700.

Report (1964) First Report of the Expert Committee on Drug Toxicity. London: Association of the British Pharmaceutical Industry.

Report (1966) Principles for pre-clinical testing of drug safety. World Health Organization Technical Report Series no. 341. Geneva: WHO.

Report (1976) Report of a European Workshop. *Eur. J. Clin. Pharmacol.* **11**, 233–238.

Report (1978) Long Term Toxic Effects. A Study Group Report. London: The Royal Society.

Weatherall, M. (1982). An end to the search for new drugs? *Nature, Lond.* **296**, 387–390.

# 2

# Bethanidine

A. F. GREEN and M. WEATHERALL
*Wellcome Research Laboratories, Beckenham, Kent, England*

## I. Summary

Bethanidine (N-benzyl-N′N′′-dimethylguanidine sulphate) is an adrenergic-neurone blocking agent introduced into the U.K. and other countries in 1964 for the treatment of hypertension. It was first synthesized in 1960 and received clinical trials from 1961 onwards, while preclinical studies were continuing. These studies consisted of acute pharmacological observations in cats, dogs and monkeys, and longer experiments with daily doses to cats and monkeys for two or six months, also to rats for up to twelve months. The acute experiments showed no important effects other than those due to adrenergic blockade. The longer experiments did not show any tissue damage attributable to the drug. No ill effects were observed on the foetuses of pregnant rats and rabbits except after doses sufficient to cause maternal deaths. Impaired fertility was shown to be due to failure of ejaculation caused by sympathetic blockade. No carcinogenic properties were found. In brief pharmacokinetic studies, the drug was found to have a selective affinity for adrenergic neurones. Some interactions were noted with catecholamines and with drugs affecting amine uptake and storage mechanisms. The blood pressure of renal hypertensive rats was reduced by the drug. Clinical use of the drug in the U.K. reached a maximum about ten years after it was introduced, with about 400,000 prescriptions issued per year. Reported adverse reactions were infrequent and most could be related to impaired autonomic function. The case history exemplifies the standards initially used by U.K. regulatory authorities. Some of the preclinical experiments were essential in selecting one compound among many candidates for trial, and the predictive value of the experiments, as far as it was tested, was good. The longer term experiments were reassuring but remain of unproven value as evidence.

## II. Introduction

During the 1950s the control of hypertension depended on the use of ganglion blocking agents. The treatment was unsatisfactory because the drugs produced parasympathetic as well as sympathetic blockade and so caused many unwanted effects. A considerable advance was made by the first introduction to medical practice of a specific adrenergic neurone blocking agent, namely, bretylium, which was synthesized and developed at the U.K. laboratories of the Wellcome Research Foundation (Boura *et al.*, 1959a, b; Boura and Green, 1959) and marketed in the United Kingdom in 1959. It was effective in clinical trials and early clinical use, but its use declined rapidly because tolerance, which had been anticipated from studies in cats (Boura *et al.*, 1959b), developed to an extent which made it inadequately effective (Dollery *et al.*, 1960; Turner, 1960; Johnston *et al.*, 1962). Also, a number of subjects developed parotid pain during treatment (Laurence and Rosenheim, 1960; Turner, 1960). At about this time guanethidine was discovered (Maxwell *et al.*, 1959, 1960) and became acknowledged to be a better drug for blocking adrenergic neurones in clinical practice. Meanwhile, the line of research which led to bretylium had been extended, and of the many compounds examined in animals (for review see Copp, 1964) five were investigated in man. Three of these are referred to in the literature (Boura, *et al.*, 1960a, 1961; Montuschi and Pickens, 1962; Boura and Green, 1963). The one which proved best, N-benzyl-N'N''-dimethylguanidine sulphate, was named bethanidine (Montuschi and Pickens, 1962; Smirk, 1963; Prichard *et al.*, 1968) and introduced into general use in the U.K. in 1964. This was the time at which

Bethanidine

Bretylium

Guanethidine

a voluntary system of control of new drugs in the U.K. (the Committee on Safety of Drugs or "Dunlop Committee") was beginning to operate, and the submission on bethanidine was among the earliest to be considered. No precedent existed, and the submission is therefore interesting as a model of the standards which were regarded as acceptable at that time. Bethanidine was marketed in many other countries, but the submission, like many other submissions, particularly on cardiovascular drugs (Wardell, 1974), was delayed by the American F.D.A. An application made by A. H. Robins and Co. in 1975 was approved only in 1981. The drug has not so far (1983) been marketed in the United States. It has remained in clinical use in other countries and, as discussed later, has a negligible record of adverse effects other than those attributable to its main pharmacological action.

## III. Preclinical and toxicological data

The laboratory data accumulated on bethanidine between the time of its discovery and the time of marketing were initially the subject of detailed internal Company reports. The first two reports, of November 1960, were provided to the original clinical investigators, and were the basis for the first trials of the compound in man. Further information was made available as it accumulated, and the complete set formed the basis of the submission to the Committee on Safety of Drugs, and the justification for initial marketing. The main pharmacological findings were subsequently published (Boura and Green, 1963; Green and Robson, 1964, 1965; for reviews see Boura and Green, 1981; Green, 1982; Maxwell and Wastila, 1977).

The summaries of the first two reports were worded as follows:

*"Summary of important biological properties*
The main action of this compound is to block adrenergic nerve mechanisms. Its effects are similar to those of guanethidine and bretylium, with both of which 467C60* has some chemical similarity. It is however more potent than either of these agents and appears to be fully absorbed from the alimentary tract. Its duration of action is similar to that of guanethidine. In acute tests in animals there is a wide margin between the dose which blocks the adrenergic mechanism and that producing toxic effects. The main toxic action appears to be paralysis of the respiration. Chronic tests have revealed no cumulative toxic action. Animals given daily injections of the drug develop some tolerance as to guanethidine and bretylium and likewise this is associated with the "denervated" smooth muscles becoming hypersensitive to noradrenaline and adrenaline".

*467C60 was the code number used at that time for bethanidine.

and

"*Summary of chronic toxicity studies*
The drug has been given daily to rats, cats and monkeys for periods of up to 2 months. The amounts given were at least 20 times the amounts causing a substantial depression of adrenergic nerve function in cats. No toxic action was apparent in rats given 10 or 50 mg/kg orally. Subcutaneous doses of 50 mg/kg retarded the growth in a a group of 5 cats, one animal dying after 2 weeks. In no instance was there evidence of tissue damage but some infiltration into the adrenal medulla was apparent in 2 animals; as such changes could not be found in rats or monkeys the significance of this finding is doubtful. There was an indication that daily administration of 50 mg/kg orally was toxic in 2 monkeys but 4 others were apparently unaffected. None of 4 monkeys given 10 mg/kg have shown adverse response during 2 months—they are being kept on the drug".

It is instructive to note the recommendations for dosage for clinical trials, which were included in the initial pharmacological report and ran as follows:

"*Recommended Dosage for Clinical Trials*
On the grounds that 467C60 sulphate is about 3 times as active as guanethidine in cats by injection and orally, we would expect the dose that will impair sympathetic activity in man to be 10–20 mg. This is also the expected effective dose from consideration of the amounts which caused some impairment of sympathetic function in cats, and dogs—these doses approximate to 0.3 mg/kg which is equivalent to 18 mg in a 60 kg man. We suggest however that no more than 5 mg should be given on the first occasion. The oral dose is likely to be similar to the injected dose.
If the drug is to be given intravenously there seems no contraindication to the amount administered being increased at intervals of 30 min. The main toxic action in cats is on breathing and this occurs with doses of about 10 mg/kg i.v. (600 mg/60 kg) and over 100 mg/kg when the drug is given subcutaneously or orally. The respiratory paralysis with an intravenous dose of 10 mg/kg in cats lasts only a few minutes and cats have been recovered from 15 mg/kg by application of artificial respiration. No necrotic action was shown by a 10 mg/ml solution when injected intradermally in guinea-pigs".

The estimates of potency and duration of action were based on studies of the relaxation of the nictitating membranes in cats caused by single subcutaneous doses. Studies of cumulative effects and of the depletion of the adrenergic transmitter had not been made at the time. It is now recognized that daily doses of guanethidine are highly cumulative in animals and rapidly cause substantial depletion of tissue amines by comparison with bethanidine (for review see Maxwell and Wastila, 1977). This probably accounts for the recovery from sympathetic blockade following a course of treatment, with bethanidine being much more rapid than after guanethidine treatment in man as in laboratory animals. In all other respects the statements provided accurate predictions relevant to the action, potency and safety of the drug in man.

At this time (1961–63) no requirement existed for official authorization of clinical trials, and these proceeded satisfactorily and promptly. More prolonged studies of toxicity in animals were proceeding at the same time, and reports on them were available at the time when the Committee on the Safety of Drugs was preparing to operate with the voluntary co-operation of the pharmaceutical industry. Summaries of two of these reports, as submitted to and used by the Committee read as follows:

## A. Chronic Toxicity Studies

"No contraindication to the use of bethanidine for controlling hypertension in man by blocking adrenergic nerves has been found in the experiments described in this report. Large doses of bethanidine have been given daily to rats for 12 months and to dogs, cats and monkeys for up to 6 months. The drug was given orally except in the cats, for which the subcutaneous route was chosen. Records were kept of growth. Haematological and clinical biochemistry examinations were carried out at intervals. At the termination of the experiment the main organs were weighed and a detailed histological study made.

Doses of up to 10 mg/kg, equivalent to about ten times the amounts required to depress sympathetic nerve function, showed no toxic effect whatsoever in any of the species used.

In the rats a lethal effect occurred occasionally soon after drug administration when the dosage was 50 mg/kg but a few animals survived 500 mg/kg daily for 12 months. No other untoward effects were observed except retardation of growth with the 500 mg/kg doses. A few organ weights showed some minor deviations from control values and in the 500 mg/kg group erythrocyte counts were slightly reduced.

No untoward effects occurred in dogs given 20–25 mg/kg bethanidine daily but growth was retarded by 80–100 mg/kg. A few minor variations in organ weights were observed. The blood picture suggested that a slight non-progressive haemodilution occurred after giving drug for a few weeks.

Subcutaneous doses of 50 mg/kg in cats were well tolerated for a period of 6 months.

All monkeys given 10 mg/kg bethanidine daily by stomach tube for 6 months and 4 of 6 given 50 mg/kg daily for 2 months were unaffected. In the group on the higher dose, one animal began to lose weight after a month and another died unexpectedly after 7 weeks. No satisfactory explanation of their illnesses were found. The examination of the tissues did not show any structural change thought to be due to drug action.

At least some of the minor organ weight variations may be attributable to adrenergic neurone blockade and some of the variations were not consistent between species".

## B. Studies in Pregnant Animals

"Daily administration of bethanidine to pregnant rats and rabbits produced no harmful effect on foetal development even when the drug was given at doses greatly exceeding those used for treating hypertension in man. When the dosage was sufficient to cause some maternal deaths and a marked reduction in weight gain, at a level of 100–200 mg/kg by stomach tube, a small but significant increase in embryonic deaths was found in rats. No contraindication to the use of bethanidine during pregnancy is suggested by these experiments".

## C. Further Studies

When male and female rats receiving approximately 50 mg/kg bethanidine daily in their diet were mated after receiving drug for 6 to 9 weeks markedly reduced fertility was found. Comment on this preliminary experiment ran as follows.

"The experiment suggests that the impairment of fertility caused by bethanidine may be due to failure of the males to impregnate the females with adequate spermatozoa. This possibility is in keeping with reports that ejaculation is suppressed by the drug in man. Like other adrenergic neurone blocking agents bethanidine apparently blocks the sympathetic mechanism on which ejaculation depends. Confirmation that this is the cause of the reduced fertility in rats on bethanidine is being sought by withdrawing the males from drug treatment. The experiment also shows that lactation is fully satisfactory in bethanidine treated animals and that the growth and development of their litters is not impaired".

A further brief report ran as follows:

"*Assessment of Carcinogenicity*
Experiments described [in an earlier report] in which large doses of bethanidine have been given daily for a year in rats and for 6 months in dogs, cats and monkeys did not reveal any carcinogenic properties.
The possibility of bethanidine having a carcinogenic action in animals is being explored further by continuing drug administration for 2 years in rats and 80 weeks in mice".

The "large doses" referred to are those described above in the paragraph headed "Chronic Toxicity", i.e. up to 500 mg/kg daily by stomach tube in rats, up to 80–100 mg/kg on five days per week orally in dogs, up to 50 mg/kg daily subcutaneously in cats and up to 10 mg/kg daily by stomach tube in monkeys.

## D. Pharmacokinetics

Observations on the distribution and excretion by cats of [14]C-labelled bethanidine had already been published in 1962 by Boura *et al.*, and formed part of the submission to the Committee on Safety of Drugs. Estimations were reported on the quantity of [14]C in twenty organs and tissues of two cats, and in nerves and ganglia from eighteen sites, together with details of urinary excretion after subcutaneous and after oral administration, each in two cats. A search for metabolites showed little evidence of chemical change *in vivo*. The selective affinity of the drug for adrenergic neurones was demonstrated.

This affinity accounted for its specificity of action, as had previously been found for bretylium (Boura *et al.*, 1960b; Green, 1960).

On this basis, bethanidine was agreed by the regulatory authority in the United Kingdom as being safe for marketing, and its use began in various countries. Toxicological studies continued, and a number of out-standing points were clarified as follows.

## E. Continuation of Reproduction Studies

As already mentioned the finding that the fertility of rats was impaired when both sexes were receiving bethanidine led to investigation of the effect of withdrawing the drug from the males only. Impairment of fertility did not persist, thus supporting the earlier supposition that the only significant adverse effect of bethanidine on reproductive processes is the expected impairment of the ejaculatory mechanism which is dependent upon sympathetic innervation.

The study of foetal development in rabbits was extended by dissection of two formalin fixed foetuses from each of 11 litters from does treated with bethanidine sulphate (150 mg/kg per day orally from days 8–16 of pregnancy) and from 2 litters of control animals run at the same time. "No abnormalities were found."

## F. French Visa

In order to obtain a "visa" for marketing in France, it was necessary to satisfy the demand for a direct comparison of the toxicity of pulverized bethanidine ("Esbatal") tablets with the pure drug by daily administration for three months in young rats. The doses of each were 10 or 50 mg/kg of active ingredient per day. No effects were discovered on weight gain, survival or behaviour. No haematological or histopathological change attributable to drug action was found.

## G. Continuation of Carcinogenicity Studies

The two studies mentioned above were carried out primarily with the objective of discovering whether malignant changes might arise as a consequence of treatment with the drug. In one the compound was given to young rats at a dose of 20 mg/kg per day for two years. In the other, 50 mg/kg of bethanidine was given daily to mice for 80 weeks. Neither study revealed an adverse effect attributable to the drug. The organs examined after completion of dosing in both studies were kidney, liver, lung, spleen, heart, brain, pituitary, adrenal, thyroid, thymus, ovary, uterus, prostate, seminal vesicle, testis, stomach, duodenum or ileum, colon, pancreas, bone marrow, skeletal muscle, salivary gland, and urinary bladder. Two blocks of brain tissue were taken and the sections were stained; stainable disulphide groups were compared with the normal, in order to detect changes in the amount of neuro-secretory material in tracts known to be influenced by catecholamines. The adrenals were examined for general morphology as well as distribution of fat and chromaffin tissue. In the pancreas $\alpha$ and $\beta$ cells were stained and compared by two techniques. The kidney, in addition to the usual haematoxylin and eosin, was stained with periodic acid Schiff and Alcian Blue. The rest of the organs were examined morphologically.

## H. Alternative Method of Manufacture

During 1967, an alternative method of manufacture was devised, which led to a product containing up to 0.75% trimethylguanidine rather than the earlier trace amounts. Studies on trimethylguanidine showed that it was substantially less toxic than bethanidine, was less effectively absorbed from the alimentary tract, and produced symptoms of much more brief duration. The impurity had weak ganglion blocking properties, and in lethal amounts caused neuromuscular paralysis. These acute pharmacodynamic studies on the compound indicated that the new method of manufacture was acceptable and were sufficient to satisfy the U.K. regulatory authority.

## I. Tests in Hypertensive Rats

The availability of an inbred strain of New Zealand hypertensive rats (Smirk, 1973) enabled studies on the effect of bethanidine against hypertension in laboratory animals:

> "Bethanidine lowered the blood pressure of renal hypertensive rats. The minimal effective dose by stomach tube is between 3 and 10 mg/kg. The effect was marked with 10 mg/kg and greater with 30 mg/kg. Doses of 100 mg/kg lowered blood pressure less than 30 mg/kg and this may be attributed to the sympathomimetic action of large amounts. Blood pressures were slightly lower with all dosages on the second than on the first day of dosing".

This study has, of course, little toxicological significance, but represents a modest improvement in laboratory procedures for predicting effects in pathological circumstances in man.

## J. Interactions with Other Drugs

Highly important interactions between the effects of bethanidine and sympathomimetic amines were expected because of the known effects of bretylium and guanethidine (Boura and Green, 1959, 1962; Green, 1960;

Maxwell *et al.*, 1960). Like the known adrenergic neurone blocking agents, bethanidine enhanced sensitivity to the directly acting amines, noradrenaline and adrenaline, in acute tests in cats (Boura and Green, 1963) and more especially when it had been given daily for a week or two when the hypersensitivity was comparable with that following postganglionic nerve section (Green and Robson, 1965). As with the earlier drugs, the extent of this hypersensitivity was greater in some effector systems, for example the nictitating membranes, than in others, including the vascular system. Like the earlier adrenergic neurone blocking agents, bethanidine could either increase or decrease responses to indirect acting amines depending upon the amount of noradrenaline released and the tissue sensitivity to that noradrenaline (Boura and Green, 1962, 1963). These observations have relevance to the possible use of some appetite suppressants and of nasal decongestants, such as dexamphetamine and ephedrine, in subjects undergoing treatment with bethanidine. Other observations are also relevant to this situation. Just as dexamphetamine powerfully antagonizes acute blockade of adrenergic neurones by bretylium and guanethidine (Day, 1962), so also it antagonizes acute blockade by bethanidine (Boura and Green, 1963) but, as also is the case with guanethidine, the antagonism was less effective after prolonged blockade by bethanidine (Follenfant and Robson, 1970). Another important interaction occurs with desmethylimipramine and related tricyclic antidepressants as they, by suppressing the amine pump, were found to interfere with the uptake and consequent effect of the adrenergic neurone blocking agents including bethanidine (Carlson and Waldeck, 1965; Mitchell, Arias and Oates, 1967; Mitchell and Oates, 1970). The sympathomimetic effects of low doses of ergotamine are attributable to adrenoceptor activation and it was therefore relevant to know whether bethanidine might enhance its effect. Some enhancement was found but this was substantially less than to adrenaline or noradrenaline, suggesting that neuronal uptake of ergotamine is small and that the use of ergotamine and bethanidine in the same patient is not contraindicated (Follenfant and Green, 1970).

Some interactions were looked for on the grounds of possible clinical importance rather than because of pharmacological considerations. These studies were the subject of an internal Wellcome report in 1969 as follows:

"Bethanidine given each day for 5 days at a dose level which lowered sympathetic tone did not alter significantly the acute toxicity in mice of suxamethonium, pethidine, ergometrine or thiopentone. Administration of single doses of bethanidine for 5 days did not alter significantly the times of induction and duration of anaesthesia in the pregnant rat or the viability of the neonates, after administration of halothane or nitrous oxide. After daily subcutaneous adrenergic neurone blocking doses of bethanidine were given for 14 days the bradycardia and hypotension caused by halothane in the decerebrate cat tended to be increased".

The synergism mentioned in this last paragraph was of course expected.

These studies completed the basic laboratory observations on bethanidine. Some observations were made in laboratories elsewhere, in relation to the requirement of overseas registration authorities. As far as we are aware, no new properties relevant to the clinical use of bethanidine were revealed in this way. Hesitations on the part of one registration authority appeared to depend on rather precise technical details of reports and the uncertain cause of death in a small number of individual rats in large studies. The relevance of such minutiae to the broad picture presented by the original studies, and particularly after several years of administration to humans, is questionable, and will not be pursued in the present report. Clinical use and adverse reactions are dealt with in the next section of this chapter.

## IV. Clinical experience

Bethanidine was approved by the U.K. regulatory authority and marketed in the U.K. as tablets of 10 mg and 50 mg under the brand name "Esbatal" in January 1964. An alternative preparation in capsules was later sold under the brand name "Bethanid." Bethanidine was registered under these or similar names in at least 52 other countries, but the amounts supplied to most of them were very small. In 1971 the main users were Japan, U.K., Australia, Sweden, New Zealand, Canada and South Africa, which collectively accounted for 99% of the manufacturer's sales of 1620 kg in that year. Sales declined considerably in the late 1970's when agents which blocked $\beta$-adrenoceptors became preferred for the treatment of hypertension.

The number of prescriptions for bethanidine issued in any country is not usually known, but figures for those prescribed by general practitioners in the National Health Service of the United Kingdom have been reported as follows: 1972—330,600; 1973—380,200; 1974—402,400; 1975—372,900.

A rough estimate of the number of patients who are likely to have received bethanidine for a year, often considerably longer, can be derived by examination of the prescriptions issued in U.K. during 1973, when the use of bethanidine was nearing its peak. From information on prescription dosages in the Medical Data Index, 1973, the 380,200 prescriptions reported by the U.K. Department of Health and Social Security represented 34,190 patient years of therapy. That number would be exceeded by the total number of patients receiving the drug in that year for two reasons. First, although treatment for hypertension is usually a continued process, some changes of the choice of drug are to be expected. The extent of such changes can be gauged from the Medical Data Index, 1973; 5% of the bethanidine prescriptions are defined as "new" and 4.3% as "switch prescriptions". Second, the above figures do not include the prescribing of bethanidine by doctors in hospitals for in-patients or more frequently for out-patients. Such prescriptions are likely to be a small but significant proportion of the total. It seems likely therefore, that the number of patients in the U.K. who received bethanidine for prolonged time periods is of the order of 40,000 but precise information is lacking.

Important though it is to estimate the size of the population at risk, it is not in this instance crucial because reports of adverse reactions were minimal. In the United Kingdom, the Committee on Safety of Medicines (the statutory successor to the voluntary Committee mentioned earlier) registered between January 1964 and February 1980 a total of 131 reports, 6 fatal, in which bethanidine was mentioned. The fatal reactions were attributed, one each, to hypertension rebound, haematemesis, hepatitis, myocardial infarction, cerebrovascular disorder and haemorrhage. The non-fatal reactions were scattered over a wide range of symptoms. The largest group of reports referred, not surprisingly, to the autonomic nervous system, with 28 instances, including seven of hypertension, five of hypotension, four of syncope, three of diarrhoea, and two each of lachrymal gland disorder, palpitation, tachycardia and vasospasm. The next largest group referred to skin disorders, over half the 20 reports being of various or unspecified rashes. As the Committee on Safety of Medicines remarked: "the inclusion of a particular reaction in the Register does not mean that it is causally related to the use of the drug", since all drugs which the patient was consuming at the time are recorded as possibly causative. In this context, reactions referred to the autonomic nervous system may reasonably be connected with the drug or the disease for which it was being used. Many of the reports related to patients being treated with several drugs, and the identity of the responsible agent was not established. The reports not referring to the autonomic nervous system are sufficiently varied and sufficiently infrequent, even with allowance for under reporting, to suggest no specific effect whatever of bethanidine beside the adrenergic blockade for which it was developed.

Additional sources of information are consistent with this conclusion. The manufacturing company in the U.K. received a total of four reports between April 1968 and April 1980 of adverse reactions in which bethanidine was a concomitant drug. Each case was substantially different from the others, and in each it seemed almost certain that the reactions were unrelated to bethanidine. Data provided by Intercontinental Medical Statistics (Australia) indicates a pattern of usage of bethanidine in Australia similar to that in the U.K. during the period 1972–1975, the total of some 206,000 prescriptions approximating to one seventh of that for the U.K. in the same period. The Australian Drug Evaluation Committee, in its fourth report published in 1978, covering the period 1964–76, recorded 16 adverse reactions to bethanidine sulphate. Six consisted of "postural hypotension", two of "hypotension" and the remaining eight were scattered over different causes. In relation to the quantity of drug supplied in Australia, the picture is essentially identical with the U.K. experience. Records from New Zealand involve still smaller numbers but follow the same pattern. For other countries, formally collected data are not at present available to us, but the absence from the world medical literature of published reports of adverse reactions does not suggest that regional problems exist which differ from those observed in the country of origin.

## V. Conclusions

The question which this account seeks to answer is "what value in preventing human illness had the toxicological studies made in animals?" Unequivocally, the pharmacological studies were essential for the selection of good candidates for trial in man. Over 400 newly synthesized compounds were available, each with some theoretical rationale, for use in the control of hypertension. Selection by experimentation in animals was inescapable. We shall probably never know for certain whether any would have been better than bethanidine, but, as already mentioned, the data from experimental animals were remarkably useful in predicting human responses, even in quite detailed matters (Prichard *et al.*, 1968; Prichard and Walden, 1979). But the value of long-term experiments, lasting for 6–12 months or more, remains unproven, although such experiments gave considerable confidence to all concerned in the use of the drug. Bethanidine was mercifully free from adverse reactions, other than those implicit in its specific phamacological property of blocking adrenergic neurones reversibly. By the standards of 1980, the initial toxicology was lacking or minimal in a variety of ways which would now be considered mandatory. The case of bethanidine is instructive particularly for historical reasons; for later developments it will be more useful to consider other drugs.

## Acknowledgements

The internal Wellcome reports forming the basis of this Chapter represent the work of several of our previous colleagues to whom we extend our thanks. Particularly major contributions to these reports were made by the late Dr. Vernon Udall who, at the time, was Head of the Department of Pathology and responsible for much of the toxicology and by Professor Alan Boura who was responsible for many of the pharmacological studies described.

# References

Boura, A. L. A. and Green, A. F. (1959) The actions of bretylium: adrenergic neurone blocking and other effects. *Br. J. Pharmacol.* **14**, 536–548.

Boura, A. L. A. and Green, A. F. (1962) Comparison of bretylium and guanethidine: Tolerance and effects on adrenergic nerve function and responses to sympathomimetic amines. *Br. J. Pharmacol.* **19**, 13–41.

Boura, A. L. A. and Green, A. F. (1963) Adrenergic neurone blockade and other acute effects caused by N-benzyl-N'N''-dimethyl guanidine and its ortho-chloro derivate. *Br. J. Pharmacol.* **20**, 36–55.

Boura, A. L. A. and Green, A. F. (1981) Adrenergic neurone blocking agents (A histological perspective). *J. Auton. Pharmacol.* **1**, 255–267.

Boura, A. L. A., Copp, F. C. and Green, A. F. (1959a) New adrenergic compounds. *Nature* **184**, B.A.70–B.A.71.

Boura, A. L. A., Green, A. F., McCoubrey, A., Laurence, D. R., Moulton, R. and Rosenheim, M. L. (1959b) Darenthin. Hypotensive agent of new type. *Lancet* **ii**, 17–21.

Boura, A. L. A., Coker, G. G., Copp, F. C., Duncombe, W. G., Elphick, A. R., Green, A. F. and McCoubrey, A. (1960a) Powerful adrenergic neurone-blocking agents related to choline 2,6-xylyl ether bromide. *Nature* **185**, 925–926.

Boura, A. L. A., Copp, F. C., Duncombe, W.G., Green, A. F. and McCoubrey, A. (1960b) The selective accumulation of bretylium in sympathetic ganglia and their post ganglionic nerves. *Br. J. Pharmacol.* **15**, 265–270.

Boura, A. L. A., Copp, F. C., Green, A. F., Hodson, H. F., Ruffell, G. K., Sim, M. F., Walton, E. and Grivsky, E. M. (1961) Adrenergic neurone-blocking agents related to choline 2,6-xylyl ether bromide (*TM*10), bretylium and guanethidine. *Nature* **191**, 1312–1313.

Boura, A. L. A., Duncombe, W. G., Robson, R. D. and McCoubrey, A. (1962) The distribution and excretion by cats of a new hypotensive drug, N-benzyl-N'N''-dimethylguanidine. *J. Pharm. Pharmacol.* **14**, 722–726.

Carlsson, A. and Waldeck, B. (1965) Mechanism of amine transport in the cell membranes of the adrenergic nerves. *Acta Pharmacol. Toxicol.* **22**, 293–300.

Copp, F. C. (1964) Adrenergic neurone blocking agents. *In:* "Advances in Drug Research", **1**, 161–189.

Day, M. D. (1962) Effect of sympathomimetic amines on the blocking action of guanethidine, bretylium and xylocholine. *Br. J. Pharmacol.* **18**, 421–439.

Dollery, C. T., Emslie-Smith, D. and McMichael, J. (1960) Bretylium tosylate in the treatment of hypertension. *Lancet* **i**, 296–299.

Follenfant, M. and Green, A. F. (1970) Effects of bethanidine on responses to ergotamine and noradrenaline. *Br. J. Pharmacol.* **39**, 225P–226P.

Follenfant, M. J. and Robson, R. D. (1970) The antagonism of adrenergic neurone blockade by amphetamine and dexamphetamine in the rat and guinea-pig. *Br. J. Pharmacol.* **38**, 792–801.

Green, A. F. (1960) The effects of bretylium and allied agents on adrenergic neurones. *In:* "Ciba Foundation Symposium on Adrenergic Mechanisms". March 28–31, London. (Vane, J. R., Wolstenholme, G. E. W., O'Connor, M. Eds.) pp. 148–157. London: Churchill.

Green, A. F. (1982) The discovery of bretylium and bethanidine. *Br. J. Clin. Pharmacol.* **13**, 25–34.

Green, A. F. and Robson, R. D. (1964) Comparison of the effects of bretylium, guanethidine and bethanidine on smooth muscle responses to different rates of sympathetic nerve stimulation. *Br. J. Pharmacol.* **22**, 349–355.

Green, A. F. and Robson, R. D. (1965) Adrenergic neuron blocking agents: tolerance and hypersensitivity to adrenaline and noradrenaline. *Br. J. Pharmacol.* **25**, 497–506.

Johnston, A. W., Prichard, B. N. C. and Rosenheim, M. L. (1962) Adrenergic neurone-blocking agents. *Lancet* **ii**, 996.

Laurence, D. R. and Rosenheim, M. L. (1960) Clinical effects of drugs which prevent the release of adrenergic transmitter. "Ciba Foundation Symposium on Adrenergic Mechanisms". March 28–31, London. (Vane, J. R., Wolstenholme, G. E. W. and O'Connor, M. Eds.) pp. 201–208. London: Churchill.

Maxwell, R. A. and Wastila, W. B. (1977) Adrenergic neurone blocking drugs. "Handbook of Experimental Pharmacology". Vol. 39: Antihypertensive agents. (Gross, F. Ed.) pp. 161–162. Berlin Heidelberg. New York. Springer-Verlag.

Maxwell, R. A., Mull, R. P. and Plummer, A. J. (1959) [2-(octahydro-1-azocinyl)-ethyl]-guanidine sulfate (CIBA 5864-SU) a new synthetic antihypertensive agent. *Experientia (Basel)* **15**, 267.

Maxwell, R. A., Plummer, A. J., Schneider, F., Povalski, H. and Daniel, A. I. (1960) Pharmacology of [2-(octahydro-1-azocinyl)-ethyl]-guanidine sulphate (SU-5864). *J. Pharmacol. exp. Ther.* **128**, 22–29.

Mitchell, J. R. and Oates, J. A. (1970) Guanethidine and related agents. I. Mechanism of the selective blockade of adrenergic neurones and its antagonism by drugs. *J. Pharmacol. exp. Ther.* **172**, 100–107.

Mitchell, J. R., Arias, L. and Oates, J. A. (1967) Antagonism of the antihypertensive action of guanethidine sulfate by desipramine hydrochloride. *J. Am. med. Ass.* **202**, 973–976.

Montuschi, E. and Pickens, P. T. (1962) A clinical trial of two related adrenergic neurone blocking agents—BW 392C60 and BW 467C60. *Lancet* **ii**, 897–901.

Prichard, B. N. C. and Walden, R. J. (1979) Some major consequences of actions of drugs on the autonomic nervous system in man and experience of prediction from animal studies. *Pharmacol. Ther.* **5**, 55–59.

Prichard, B. N. C., Johnston, A. W., Hill, I. D. and Rosenheim, M. L. (1968) Bethanidine, guanethidine, and methyldopa in the treatment of hypertension: a within-patient comparison. *Br. med. J.* **1**, 135–144.

Smirk, F. H. (1963) The hypotensive action of BW 476C60. *Lancet* **i**, 743–746.

Smirk, F. H. (1973) Experimental Genetic Hypertension. *In:* "Hypertension: Mechanisms and Management". (Onesti, G., Kim, K. E., and Moyer, J. H., Eds.) pp. 59–65. New York and London: Grune & Stratton.

Turner, R. W. D. (1960) Bretylium. "Ciba Foundation Symposium on Adrenergic Mechanisms". March 28–31, London (Vane, J. R., Wolstenholme, G. E.W. and O'Connor, M. Eds.) pp. 209–212. London: Churchill.

Wardell, W. M. (1974) Therapeutic implications of the drug lag. *Clin. Pharmacol. Ther.* **15**, 73–96.

# 3

# Bromocriptine

B. P. RICHARDSON[1], I. TURKALJ[2], E. FLÜCKIGER[1]

[1] *Preclinal Research Department and* [2] *Drug Monitoring Centre, Pharmaceutical Division, Sandoz Ltd., CH-4002 Basel, Switzerland*

## I. Summary

The search for an ergot compound which selectively and potently inhibited pituitary prolactin secretion started in 1962. 2-Br-$\alpha$-ergokryptine (bromocriptine, CB 154) was first synthesized in 1965 and by the end of 1967 had been shown to inhibit prolactin-dependent phenomena in animals (implantation of fertilized ova in the rat, lactation in several species). Importantly, it lacked the prominent uterotonic and pressor activities characteristic of so many ergot compounds. Although prolactin was not then recognized as a distinct entity in humans, it was nevertheless decided to test bromocriptine's ability to suppress lactation in humans. The initial animal toxicity studies (acute toxicity in mice, rats and rabbits, four week oral toxicity studies in dogs and rats, and a teratology study in rats) were designed so as to permit multiple oral dosing in women of childbearing age. The results revealed no findings which were prohibitive to the clinical testing of bromocriptine in humans. Preliminary clinical studies were completed by August 1971 and showed that bromocriptine was both well tolerated and effective in inhibiting puerperal and non-puerperal lactation. During these studies it was also shown that some women with amenorrhoea and galactorrhoea started to menstruate again and became fertile. At about this time the presence of prolactin in man was identified and a radioimmunoassay for its measurement in serum samples became available.

Continuing animal pharmacological studies designed to elucidate the mechanism whereby it inhibits prolactin secretion showed bromocriptine to possess potent central dopaminergic activity and thus provided the rationale for investigating its efficacy in Parkinson's disease and acromegaly. However, the available animal toxicity data were not sufficient to support the long term clinical trials required to establish bromocriptine's usefulness and safety in these indications, and the treatment of infertility in women carried with it the distinct likelihood that bromocriptine administration would occur during the critical organogenetic phases of early pregnancy. Consequently it was decided to extend the existing animal toxicity data by performing a one year oral toxicity study in dogs and rats, a 13 week oral study in monkeys, teratology studies in rats and rabbits, and a fertility study in female rats.

The results obtained from these studies reflected the known pharmacological actions of the compound (dopaminergic effects or consequent inhibition of prolactin secretion). Cleft palates, which were observed in a few fetuses from mother rabbits treated with bromocriptine, only occurred at doses which were clearly toxic, or even lethal, to the dams. This effect could not be reproduced in a second breed of rabbit.

Hyperplastic, metaplastic and inflammatory changes that occurred in the uteri of female rats treated with bromocriptine for one year were shown to result from the effects of reduced prolactin secretion superimposed on the waning endocrine system which is characteristic of aging rats. They do not occur in other species, including man. These extended animal toxicity studies thus revealed no effects which spoke against further clinical testing, and during the period 1972–1976 bromocriptine emerged as first-line therapy for prolactin secreting pituitary adenomas, acromegaly, inhibition of post partum and post abortion lactation, post partum mammary congestion, incipient puerperal mastitis, galactorrhoea with or without amenorrhoea, prolactin-dependent premenstrual symptoms, prolactin-dependent menstrual disorders and subfertility, prolactin-dependent male hypogonadism, impotence and oligospermia and Parkinsonism.

Bromocriptine was first registered and marketed in 1975 for the prevention of post partum and post abortion lactation as well as for the suppression of established lactation in South Africa, Switzerland and Britain. To permit world-wide registration and marketing of bromocriptine for the other indications listed above, many of which require long-term or even life-time therapy, animal tests to investigate the carcinogenic potential of bromocriptine in rats and mice were initiated in 1975, as were additional reproduction studies (including primate teratology) and a series of mutagenicity studies. The only study that produced untoward findings was the rat carcinogenicity study, where the uterine findings observed after one year's administration of bromocriptine had progressed to neoplasia. A series of special studies showed that this is a simple manifestation of prolonged estrogen dominance brought about by the prolactin inhibitory effects of bromocriptine superimposed on the waning endocrine system of the aging female rat. It was clear to us at Sandoz as well as to the Drug Regulatory Authorities and their scientific consultants that these findings were not relevant for the human situation. Clinical experience has shown this interpretation to be correct.

Side effects have not been a major problem in humans and no fatal reactions have occurred. The most commonly observed adverse reactions are nausea and vomiting and postural hypotension. These and other minor reactions can usually be overcome by giving small initial doses of bromocriptine. Most importantly there is no evidence from the 1400 pregnancies so far monitored that bromocriptine has adverse effects on fetal development in humans. Unlike the situation observed in rats, the endometrial histology of women taking high doses of bromocriptine for long periods of time is completely normal. Digital vasospasm has been observed in acromegalic patients with a history of Raynaud's disease and who received high doses of bromocriptine. This effect disappears when the dosage is reduced. In Parkinson's disease visual hallucinations have been reported in some patients and dyskinesias similar to those observed with L-DOPA can occur in the advanced stages of the disease. These effects are believed to reflect the central dopaminergic action of the compound.

No serious clinical interactions of bromocriptine with other drugs have been reported. The monitoring and investigation of clinical adverse reactions continues, even though bromocriptine is now on the market.

An analysis of the value of the animal tests conducted with bromocriptine in predicting the presence or absence of side effects in man shows that these studies were, indeed, very useful. Although the animal toxicity tests took more than 10 years to complete at a 1982 cost of 2.7 million Swiss francs, there can be no doubt that the human benefit derived from bromocriptine fully justifies the expenditure.

## II. Introduction

Bromocriptine (2-Br-α-ergokryptine, CB 154) is an ergot compound which attracts considerable attention, both clinically and preclinically, since it is the first of a new therapeutic group of drugs, the directly acting dopaminomimetics. The availability of bromocriptine for clinical trials coincided with the start of the *Human Prolactin Era* (Editorial, 1971), and its efficacy in inhibiting non-puerperal lactation and postpartum lactation and in lowering serum prolactin levels was demonstrated shortly afterwards. At about the same time the drug was shown to stimulate dopamine receptors. This novel pharmacodynamic property subsequently led to the discovery of its beneficial effects in Parkinson's disease and of its growth hormone lowering action in acromegalic patients. The shaping of the pharmacological and therapeutic profile of bromocriptine over the past ten years and important developments in the clinical and preclinical sciences have been mutually linked, so that bromocriptine has both contributed as an investigational tool and benefited from the explosion of knowledge in the prolactin and dopamine receptor fields during this period.

The mesylate salt of bromocriptine was first marketed in 1975 and is now available under the names Parlodel® and Pravidel® in more than 100 countries for some or all of the following indications: prolactin secreting pituitary adenomas; acromegaly; post partum and post abortion lactation; post partum mammary congestion; incipient puerperal mastitis; galactorrhoea with or without amenorrhoea; prolactin-dependent premenstrual symptoms; prolactin-dependent menstrual disorders and subfertility; prolactin-dependent male hypogonadism; impotence and oligospermia; and Parkinsonism.

## III. Animal Studies

## A. The Unfolding of the Pharmacodynamic Profile

When Shelesnyak first reported in 1954 that certain ergot alkaloids suppressed luteal function and ovum implantation by reducing prolactin secretion in rats, this observation did not immediately catch the interest of pharmacologists. We first started active research in this field in 1962, when Zeilmaker and Carlsen (1962) demonstrated a direct action of such compounds on the pituitary. We wanted to know whether this new property of ergot alkaloids was linked to the other, better studied, actions, such as vasopressor, uterotonic, $\alpha$-adrenoceptor and serotonin receptor blocking activities. In particular we were interested to see whether an ergot compound could be found which inhibited prolactin secretion as its main action. We found 2-Br-$\alpha$-ergokryptine methane sulphonate (CB 154, bromocriptine mesylate), which was first synthesized in 1965 (Schneider et al., 1977), to be the most potent inhibitor of ovum implantation, and the most suitable compound in other respects (Fig. 1): it had much less pressor activity in the pithed rat than the parent compound $\alpha$-ergokryptine, no uterotonic activity, and its actions on cardiovascular parameters in anesthetized animals were not unfavourable. It was also less emetic in the dog than, for instance, ergotamine. Apart from this it seemed very important to us that bromocriptine, in contrast to natural congeners, had no late effect on the fetuses in those rats in which it did not prevent ovum implantation (Flückiger, 1972) when injected on the fifth day after insemination.

In 1967 it was decided to test bromocriptine in man as a prolactin secretion inhibitor. At that time the physiological and pharmacological state of information about prolactin was most unsuitable for such a venture. The existence of this hormone in man was generally negated (see Geschwind, 1972, and Pasteels, 1973), with the important exception of J. L. Pasteels in Brussels, whose positive evidence for the existence of human prolactin made

2-Br-α-ergokryptine-mesylate
CB 154
DCI: Bromocriptine
Parlodel®, Pravidel®

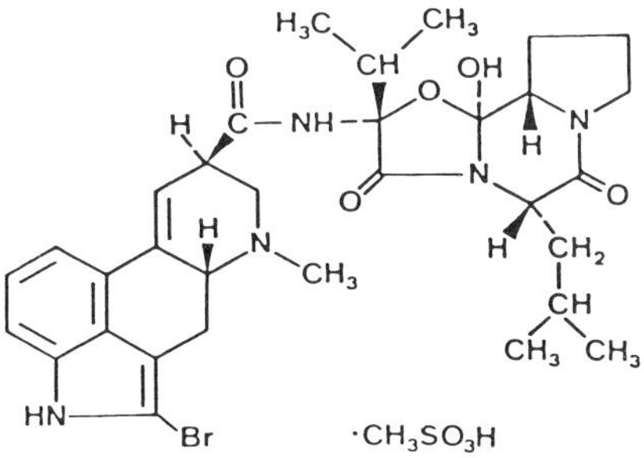

FIG. 1. Molecular structure of bromocriptine (2-Br-α-ergokryptine).

us confident for the future of the project. There existed no method to measure circulating prolactin in laboratory animals. Prolactin secretion inhibition was therefore assessed indirectly, using such indicators as those originally described by Shelesnyak in rats, as well as lactation inhibition in various species (for review see Flückiger, 1978). For clinical testing we put forth the hypothesis that prolactin was also essential for lactation in man, so that the drug should inhibit physiological and pathological lactation. Whilst studying the prolactin lowering effects of bromocriptine in patients with prolactin secreting pituitary adenomas it became evident that treatment also reduced tumor size (Corenblum *et al.*, 1975; Landolt, *et al.*, 1978; Thorner *et al.*, 1980; Wass *et al.*, 1979). This added a valuable alternative to the surgical and radiotherapeutic treatment of prolactinoma (Flückiger *et al.*, 1982).

To expand our knowledge of the pharmacodynamics of bromocriptine, the drug was given to certain leading researchers from 1969 onwards (Fuxe in Stockholm; Meites in East Lansing, Nagasawa in Tokyo; and Pasteels in Brussels). In particular they were asked questions concerning the mode of action of the drug. Their answers soon indicated that bromocriptine inhibited prolactin release from rat and human pituitaries incubated *in vitro* (Pasteels *et al.*, 1971), reduced pituitary prolactin content in mice after prolonged treatment without affecting growth hormone content (Yanai and Nagasawa, 1970, 1974), and actually reduced neurotransmitter turnover in the rat hypothalamic and neostriatal dopamine neurons. The latter observations led to the conclusion that bromocriptine was a centrally acting dopaminomimetic agent (Hökfelt and Fuxe, 1972; Corrodi *et al.*, 1973). This added dopamine receptor stimulation to the spectrum of pharmacological activities already known to exist among ergot compounds, and opened a whole new field of neuropharmacological investigation, the clinical relevance of which was soon demonstrated in patients with Parkinson's disease (Calne *et al.*, 1974a). On the basis of its dopamine agonist action, bromocriptine·was also tested in acromegalic patients and was found to reduce the concentration of growth hormone in plasma like L-DOPA, although its duration of action was much longer (Liuzzi *et al.*, 1974). In acromegalic patients and more so in patients suffering from Parkinson's disease, bromocriptine was given in higher doses than those used to reduce serum prolactin levels. Daily doses in excess of 100 mg were given over prolonged periods of time in individual cases (Thorner *et al.*, 1975b).

The introduction, at the beginning of the nineteen-seventies, of the dopamine agonist concept as the basic pharmacodynamic property of bromocriptine also greatly stimulated pre-clinical research. This resulted in a very detailed picture (Thorner *et al.*, 1980) of the interactions of bromocriptine with dopamine-sensitive functions of the CNS (Loew *et al*, 1976; Flückiger and Vigouret, 1981) and the cardiovascular and other autonomic systems. In 1976 it became established that hormone secretion from prolactin cells was mainly controlled through inhibitory dopamine receptors (MacLeod, 1976), this mechanism explaining how bromocriptine directly suppresses prolactin release. Only quite recently has it become clear that the same activation of dopamine receptors which is responsible for inhibiting prolactin secretion also suppresses the formation of prolactin messenger RNA (Maurer, 1980, 1981). This accounts for the inhibition of hormone synthesis caused by bromocriptine. Similarly, several years elapsed before the involvement of dopamine receptor interactions (pre- and postjunctional) in the cardiovascular changes produced after bromocriptine injection into anesthetized animals (the long lasting blood pressure decrease and bradycardia) was assessed (Clark *et al.*, 1978; Scholtysik, 1980; Clark, 1981). No clear effects due to $\alpha$-adrenergic or serotonin receptor interactions were seen in these studies.

Thus, today bromocriptine is characterized as a dopaminomimetic drug, and the various indications for which it is used clinically can be satisfactorily linked to this basic pharmacodynamic property.

# B. Animal Toxicity Data

## 1. Preclinical Toxicity Tests

### (a) Background
As already mentioned, it was decided in 1967 to test bromocriptine

clinically in man. Since prolactin was not yet recognized as a distinct entity in humans at that time, the most direct way of testing for suppression of prolactin in humans was to study the effects of bromocriptine on puerperal and pathological lactation in women. However, before testing in patients could begin, it was necessary to demonstrate adequate tolerance in healthy volunteers. These studies were to be conducted in Austria, Belgium, Spain and Switzerland and, although it was not required to seek approval of animal toxicity data from the respective Drug Regulatory Authorities prior to conducting such clinical studies, the battery of animal toxicity tests performed was, in fact, very similar to that required nowadays for approval from the U.S.A. or British Authorities. They were designed so as to permit limited multiple oral dosing in women of childbearing age and comprised acute toxicity studies in mice, rats and rabbits, 4 weeks oral toxicity studies in dogs and rats and a teratology study in rats.

*(b) Acute Toxicity Tests\**

"The calculated $LD_{50}$ values after observation periods of 24 h and 7 days were identical (i.e. no animals died later than 24 h after drug administration). It was only possible to calculate an oral $LD_{50}$ for mice, and even here the limits of confidence had to be extrapolated since, at the highest dose that it was possible to administer, mortality was only 80%. In rats and rabbits no deaths occurred at the highest dose possible (2000 and 1000 mg/kg respectively).

"Following intravenous administration, initial signs of toxicity were dyspnoea and motor excitation, gradually leading to rhythmic cramps, slowing respiration and coma. Similar signs were elicited by oral administration, but the rapidity of their sequence was reduced. Necropsy was done on all test animals, and revealed no unusual findings".

These studies showed that bromocriptine has a relatively high $LD_{50}$ value (>2000 mg/kg for rats and mice, >1000 mg/kg for rabbits) after oral administration in all three species. The $LD_{50}$ values obtained after intravenous injection were: mouse 190 mg/kg, rat 72 mg/kg and rabbit 12.5 mg/kg. Thus the rabbit was about 15 times more sensitive than the mouse, which is typical for ergot compounds generally.

*(c) 4 Week Oral Toxicity Studies in Rats and Dogs*

*(i) Rats* "Administration of CB154† was considered to be responsible for the following effects: excitability (agitation), hairloss and diuresis at doses of 30 and 100 mg/kg/day, dose-dependent impairment of weight gain (minimal

---

*Throughout this chapter, text within quotation marks is a citation from the original documents which were submitted by Sandoz Ltd. to the Drug Regulatory Authorities.

†CB-154 was the Sandoz code number which was used for bromocriptine at that time.

with 10 mg/kg/day, weight loss with 100 mg/kg/day), penile or clitoral erection in several rats with 30 or 100 mg/kg/day, atrophy of testicular germinal epithelium with impaired spermiogenesis at doses of 30 and 100 mg/kg/day. All other findings are considered to be secondary to these effects, or coincidental in nature. Microscopic findings in the skin in several animals are thus regarded as being a secondary response to trauma following hair loss. No specific organ toxicity, apart from that in the testes, was detected in this study. Minor increases in relative organ weights merely reflected loss in body weight at the dosage levels concerned. 10 mg/kg/day can be regarded as an oral no-toxic-effect level for the rat based on the results obtained in this study".

Since the anticipated clinical dose was about 50 times lower than this, the results observed at the 30 and 100 mg/kg/day dose levels were not considered relevant. Nevertheless, with the benefit of hindsight, we now know that hair loss, diuresis and the testicular effects are likely to be manifestations of extreme prolactin suppression in this species (Rennels and Callahan, 1959; Hafiez *et al.*, 1972; Richardson, 1973).

*(ii) Dogs.* "Administration of CB 154 to dogs was held responsible for the following effects: occasional vomiting, slight sedation, excessive salivation, and prolapse of nictitating membranes at all three dosage levels (1, 4 and 16 mg/kg/day) without obvious dose-dependence, slight dose-dependent weight loss associated with diminished food intake in the first week, followed by recovery, minor non-specific changes (thymus involution, increased fattiness of femoral bone marrow, increased lipochrome in Kupffer cells of liver and renal tubule cells) in one or more treated dogs, showing a slight degree of dose-dependence.

"All other findings are considered to be coincidental to drug administration. The elevated serum glutamic-pyruvic transaminase (SGPT) level in the female of the low level group was not accompanied by microscopic evidence of hepatotoxicity, and SGPT results at the higher dosages were normal. One high dose dog had a raised blood urea nitrogen (BUN) level, but here again histology, urinalysis and serum electrolyte results gave no indication of a nephrotoxic drug effect. No distinct target organ for CB 154 was revealed by this study. 4 mg/kg/day may be considered a non-toxic dosage level in dogs".

*(d) A Teratology Study in Rats*

"Three groups of inseminated rats (Sandoz closed breed) were treated orally, at dose levels of 3, 10 and 30 mg/kg, once a day during the organogenetic phase of gestation [days 6 to 15 *post coitum* (p.c.)]. Two additional groups were tested where the animals received a single dose of 10 mg/kg during the implantation phase on day 5 p.c. The test agent was administered by gavage, in 2% gelatine solution. A control group received plain gelatine solution in like amounts and manner as the first three groups. The parameters pertaining to the dams and fetuses were evaluated statistically. None of the investigated parameters gave evidence of any specific embryotoxic effect of the test agent.

"With a single dose of 10 mg/kg on day 5 p.c. the rate of sternal abnormalities was slightly increased and nidation was inhibited in about 30% of rats. Nidation was also inhibited in over 90% of rats with 30 mg/kg given once daily from day 6 to 15. The rate of abnormalities was not increased by repeated administrations".

The inhibition of nidation (or implantation) observed in this rat study was to be expected on the basis of bromocriptine's ability to inhibit prolactin secretion, since the maintenance of functional corpora lutea and hence implantation in this species is a prolactin dependent phenomenon. In women it is dependent on luteinizing hormone (LH), so that the effects observed in rats were not considered relevant for the clinical use of the compound. In fact subsequent clinical experience demonstrated that bromocriptine improves luteal function in hyperprolactinemic women (Del Pozo et al., 1976; Del Pozo and Lancranjan, 1978) and consequently restores menstrual cycles with ovulation. The outcome of pregnancies in such women who continued taking bromocriptine was, indeed, uneventful (Griffith et al., 1978; Turkalj et al., 1982).

Thus these initial animal toxicity studies revealed no findings which were prohibitive for the clinical testing of bromocriptine in man. Preliminary double blind tolerance and efficacy studies were completed by August 1971 and showed that bromocriptine was both well tolerated and effective in suppressing puerperal and non-puerperal lactation at doses of 3 mg t.i.d. and 5 mg t.i.d. Nausea and vomiting occurred in a few women receiving the higher dose schedule, side effects which were predictable from the findings in the four week dog oral toxicity study. Hypotensive episodes were also observed in a few patients receiving the higher dose, but no counterpart of this had been observed in previous pharmacological tests. The first reports of the clinical efficacy of bromocriptine in puerperal and non-puerperal lactation appeared in the literature shortly afterwards (Lutterbeck et al., 1971; Varga et al., 1972; Brun del Re et al., 1973).

## 2. Extended Animal Toxicity Tests

### (a) Background

In the light of the encouraging initial results, it was decided to extend the clinical trials for lactation inhibition in order to establish the optimal dosage and duration of treatment as well as efficacy against standard therapy (estrogens) in a double blind situation. Human pharmacokinetic and metabolism studies were also planned for this phase. Since early studies had shown that milk production and breast engorgement in women with non-puerperal lactation (galactorrhoea) returned promptly on withdrawing bromocriptine therapy, it became obvious that extended or even permanent medication might be required in such cases. Moreover, some women started menstruating again and it was likely that they might also ovulate and become pregnant. Clearly the animal toxicity data available at that time was inadequate for extended clinical trials, so it was decided to perform additional animal studies. Some of these clinical trials were conducted in Britain and the U.S.A., where animal toxicity test requirements were practically formalized and where prior approval of toxicity data by the Drug Regulatory Authorities was required before testing could begin. With all these considerations in mind, it was decided to extend the existing animal toxicity data by performing a one year oral toxicity study in dogs and rats, a teratology study in a second species (rabbit) and a fertility study in female rats. With the exception of the one year rat study, which was started much earlier than the other studies, they were conducted using the micronized form of the drug that was to be used clinically. Because of the improved bioavailability and increased toxicity which resulted, the doses had to be set lower than in the original 4 week studies.

An additional 13 week oral rat study was performed with one dose level of micronized drug to demonstrate the validity of the one year study with the non-micronized form. The original rat teratology study also had to be repeated using the micronized form. Because excessive vomiting occurred in dogs given this new form, even at relatively low dose levels (a typical problem with ergot compounds in this species), a 13 week oral study in rhesus monkeys was performed in addition (i.e. in a species which does not vomit so readily and is thus probably more relevant for the human situation).

*(b) A 53-Week Oral Toxicity Study in Rats*
"CB 154 was given to albino rats mixed in their feed at three dose levels—5, 20 and 82 mg/kg/day—for 53 weeks. Control rats received unmedicated feed. Extra groups of rats at the mid- and high-dose level were examined after a five-week 'recovery' period at the end of the 53 weeks, during which they received unmedicated feed.

"5 mg/kg/day was associated with slightly increased weight gain in males, decreased weight gain in females. No in-life drug effects were noted, but post mortem revealed increased adrenal weights and decreased pituitary weights in females. An increase in the number of cystic follicles with decreased luteal tissue in the ovaries, associated with some squamous metaplasia of the endometrium, indicated a drug effect on the pituitary-gonadal axis, resulting in a picture of estrogen dominance. There was apparent improvement in the severity of spontaneous interstitial nephritis in males, compared with the controls, which could possibly be attributed to a prolactin-inhibiting drug effect.

"20 mg/kg/day caused slight excitability, the same effects on weight gain as with the low-dose level, and in 2/30 blue discoloration of the tip of the tail, first seen after 37 weeks. Urinalysis revealed some evidence of diuresis, and again at this dose level there was an improvement in interstitial nephritis over that seen in the controls. Increased numbers of abnormal corpora lutea and cystic follicles in the ovaries, associated with pyometra or endometritis again suggested the picture of estrogen dominance with this dose level. 82 mg/kg/day produced similar, but more pronounced, changes to those seen with the mid-dose level. In addition, epileptiform convulsions on handling were seen in 6/13 females after 45 weeks drug administration. There was slight leucopenia, and the microscopic findings in the ovaries and uterus were more pronounced in an estrogen direction. Examination of the 'recovery' rats after a 5-week drug-free period revealed almost complete reversal of all morphologic changes.

"The presence of cystic follicles and corresponding estrogen-induced endometrial changes were not predictable on the basis of the selective prolactin-inhibiting action which CB 154 possesses. However, basic knowledge of the action of CB 154 is derived from studies made on animals with fully active endocrine systems. The findings in this prolonged oral toxicity study must therefore be considered against a background of a spontaneously declining endocrine activity, with consequent regression of ovarian function and pituitary regulation. The presence of follicular cysts and endometrial hyperplasia in the control rats of this study indicated that this was the case. The fact that cystic follicles and estrogen-induced endometrial changes were not found in rats medicated with 19 mg/kg/day CB 154 orally for 13 weeks (see p. 32) also confirms that such effects result, not from the oral administration of CB 154 *per se*, but from the effects of medication superimposed on a waning endocrine system. The effects on the female sex organs and the kidneys in this study were regarded as being pharamacodynamic rather than toxic in nature. Therefore 5 mg/kg/day can be regarded as an oral 'no-toxic effect' level for the rat".

The long term administration of bromocriptine as employed in this study revealed two new aspects, namely the ability of the drug to prevent spontaneous renal disease in rats, and the induction of ovario-uterine morphology indicative of estrogen : progesterone imbalance in rats with a waning endocrine system. Both findings were considered important enough to pursue further and were the subject of extensive investigation. The results of these studies showed that the ability of bromocriptine to prevent spontaneous renal disease in this species (see Fig. 2) relates to its prolactin

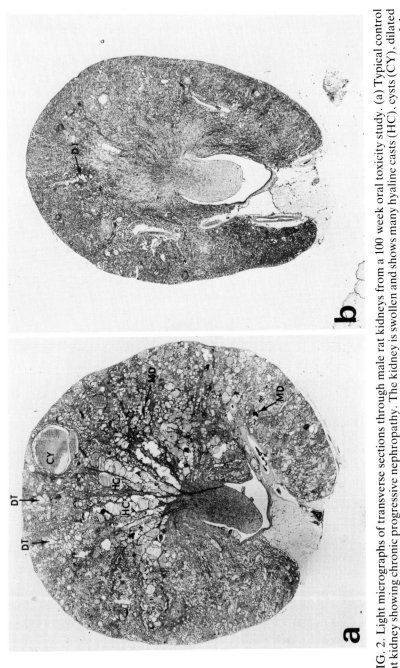

FIG. 2. Light micrographs of transverse sections through male rat kidneys from a 100 week oral toxicity study. (a) Typical control rat kidney showing chronic progressive nephropathy. The kidney is swollen and shows many hyaline casts (HC), cysts (CY), dilated tubules (DT) and mineral deposits (MD). (b) Kidney of a rat treated with 1.8 mg/kg/day bromocriptine. The appearance of the kidney is normal apart from the presence of occasional dilated tubuli (DT). Hematoxylin and eosin staining (×10).

inhibiting activity, chronic exogenous prolactin administration actually precipitating this condition (Richardson and Luginbühl 1976). These findings implicate endogenous prolactin in the etiology of degenerative renal disease in rats and their relevance for humans is currently under investigation.

Since experiments in ovariectomized rats showed that bromocriptine lacks intrinsic estrogenic activity, a series of studies aimed at elucidating the mechanism whereby chronic bromocriptine treatment induces a state of estrogen dominance were performed. They showed that although young treated female rats continued to display regular 4–5 day estrous cycles for several months (as indicated by changes in vaginal cytology), older rats (8–9 months old) showed a picture of constant estrus (vaginal cornification) within a few weeks of starting drug administration.

In contrast, age-matched controls for the latter group showed the prolonged periods of diestrus which are characteristic of pseudopregnancy. Pseudopregnancy is a common condition in older rats and occurs because normally inactive cyclical corpora lutea become activated (i.e. synthesize and secrete progesterone) by an inappropriately high circulating concentration of prolactin (Meites *et al.*, 1976). Hyperprolactinemia apparently occurs because of an age-related hypothalamic regulatory defect. It is clear that this condition cannot occur in bromocriptine treated rats because prolactin secretion is inhibited.

Although bromocriptine treatment in old pseudopregnant rats promptly initiates regular cyclical activity, this is short lived since the endocrine status of old rats is characterized not only by hypersecretion of prolactin, but also by a marked reduction in the amount of LH released during the preovulatory surge (Meites *et al.* 1976; Lu *et al.*, 1977). The consequence of this is ovulatory failure as evidenced by the presence of small cystic follicles in the ovaries and the absence of luteal tissue. Measurements of serum progesterone and estradiol levels in groups of old pseudopregnant and bromocriptine-treated rats confirmed the presence of considerably higher progesterone levels in the former group whereas estradiol levels were similar. Thus ovulation failure does not lead to elevated estradiol levels *per se,* but is associated with a higher estradiol to progesterone ratio than occurs in pseudopregnant controls. After several months this results in morphological manifestation of estrogen dominance in the genital tract, namely squamous metaplasia and endo-pyometritis.

From this series of investigations it was obvious that the ovario-uterine findings from the 53-week oral rat study were very likely to be species-specific and thus irrelevant for the clinical usage of bromocriptine. Similar findings could not be produced in a 62 week dog study (see p. 32) or in a study where mice were treated for their entire life-time with high doses (see

p. 40). More importantly, subsequent clinical studies showed that bromo-criptine did not influence follicle stimulating hormone (FSH), LH, estradiol or progesterone levels in 90 hyperprolactinemic women or in 19 menopausal acromegalic women. Moreover, endometrial biopsies in 88 patients treated with bromocriptine for 2 to 72 months at doses of 1.25 to 60 mg/day did not show any drug-related changes (Besser *et al.*, 1977).

The epileptiform convulsions that occurred on handling in 6/13 females after 45 weeks treatment with 82 mg/kg/day bromocriptine reflect central stimulatory effects which are only observed at extremely high (toxic) doses. They were not seen in males because they received a somewhat lower dose of bromocriptine (the same drug–feed mixture was used for both sexes; since females eat more relative to their body weight than do males, their drug intake was higher: males 66.2 mg/kg/day; females 97.7 mg/kg/day). Convulsions were not seen in either sex when treated with doses up to 44.5 mg/kg/day mixed in the feed for 100 weeks (see p. 37).

### (c) A Limited 13 Week Oral Study in the Rat Using the Micronized Form of Bromocriptine

"Rats were given micronized CB 154 in their feed for 13 weeks at a dose equivalent to 19 mg/kg/day (corresponding closely to the mid-level dose—20 mg/kg/day—of the 53-week study, using non-micronized drug, previously reported). The findings correspond closely with those obtained in the 53-week study with non-micronized drug (making allowances for differences in the duration of the studies). It may be concluded therefore that the results of the 53-week toxicity study in rats using non-micronized drug are valid for the micronized form".

In this study there were no cystic follicles or estrogen-induced endometrial changes observed in treated rats.

### (d) A 62-Week Oral Toxicity Study in Dogs

"CB 154 (micronized) was given orally in gelatin capsules once daily to dogs, 7 days a week for 62 weeks. Initial doses were small (0.1 mg/kg/day) because of emesis, but these were escalated over the first 10 weeks, so that for a period of 52 weeks dosage levels were 1, 3 and 10 mg/kg/day.

"During the ten-week period of escalating doses, the following changes were observed: excessive salivation, impaired food intake and weight gain (amounting to weight loss in some dogs), slightly decreased hemoglobin values associated with increased sedimentation rates and mild functional ECG changes.

"Vomiting during this period was fairly intense immediately following each increase in dose level, and the above findings are considered to be secondary to the emetic effect. The following effects continued or emerged during the period of full dosage: slight mydriasis, slight sedation, slight prolapse of nictitating membranes, sporadic dacryorrhea, superficial epithelial necrosis of dependent ear margins (self-limiting, seen with 3 and 10 mg/kg/day), increased melanin deposition in the sexual skin, impaired hair growth, slight increase in urinary specific gravity, small cystic follicles and poorly-formed or cystic corpora lutea in the ovaries, morphological evidence of thyroid over-activity, as well as non-specific pathologic changes in various organs with 10 mg/kg/day. The above changes are all considered to be an expression of exaggerated pharmacodynamic effects, or non-specific effects of over-dosage. The post mortem findings described were not seen in extra dogs allowed an eight-week 'recovery' period without medication, except for the increased pigmentation of sexual skin and hair loss in one dog. No specific organ toxic effects of CB 154 were encountered. The small necrotic lesions of the ear margin epithelium are characteristic of overdosage with ergot derivatives in dogs with low-hanging external ears, and clearly represent a trophic response to a drug effect on the vasculature at an extremely sensitive site".

In this study excessive vomiting was much more of a problem than in the original four week study. This probably occurred because the micronized form of bromocriptine was used in the 62 week study, the smaller particle size resulting in improved oral bioavailability of the compound.

Increased melanin deposition in the sexual skin is known to accompany hormonal imbalance in dogs (Muller and Kirk, 1969). The changes in ovaries suggested a prolonged drug effect on the endocrine system; corresponding changes were not seen in male gonads. None of these findings were considered relevant for humans as, indeed, clinical experience has subsequently shown. The impaired hair growth probably again reflects inhibited prolactin secretion (Rennels and Callahan, 1959), and has also been seen on rare occasions in humans treated with bromocriptine. It is reversible after discontinuing the drug treatment in both animals and humans.

*(e) 13-Week Oral Toxicity Study in Rhesus Monkeys*
"CB 154 (micronized) was given as a suspension in tragacanth by gavage to rhesus monkeys, 7 days a week, for 13 weeks. The doses used were 2, 8 and 32 mg/kg/day. 2 mg/kg/day produced slight excitability on the first 2 days of medication but thereafter no abnormal signs were observed, and all in-life examinations and post mortem studies revealed no drug-related effects. (Slight weight loss was seen in 2/4 monkeys in this and other dosage groups, including the controls, during the early weeks of the study; this is attributed to the slight stress associated with daily gavage procedure.) 8 mg/kg/day caused excitability during the first four weeks of the study. There was a slight decrease in splenic weights, but otherwise no in-life or post mortem changes attributable to a drug effect.

"32 mg/kg/day caused excitability throughout the study. There was slight weight loss in two monkeys throughout the administration period (and in the other 2 during the early weeks). Slight anemia developed in 1/4 monkeys at week 13. Splenic weights were decreased, and some swollen basophils in the anterior pituitaries of 2/4 monkeys were found.

No specific toxic effects of CB 154 emerged in this study. The pituitary findings may represent a prolactin-inhibitory drug effect. 8 mg/kg/day can be regarded as an oral 'no-toxic effect' level for the rhesus monkey".

This study demonstrated the excellent overall tolerance of bromocriptine in a species which, because of its endocrine status, was considered more relevant for the human than rats or dogs. In particular neither vomiting nor effects on the ovaries or uterus occurred.

### (f) Teratology Studies in Rats

"CB 154 was given to pregnant rats at three dose levels—3, 10 and 30 mg/kg/day—from days 6–15 *post coitum* in 1 study, and from days 8–15 *post coitum* in a second study. The drug was administered in 2% gelatin by gavage, controls receiving plain gelatin. The dams were sacrificed at term and examined together with their fetuses, maternal and fetal parameters being evaluated statistically.

"In both studies CB 154 demonstrated no embryolethal or teratogenic effect at any of the dose levels used. In the first study, where drug administration was begun during the period of implantation, inhibition of implantation was encountered with 10 and 30 mg/kg/day. Because this effect could not be demonstrated when drug administration was begun later (day 8 *post coitum*) or when it was given to rabbits during the period of implantation at the same doses (see below), it is most probably attributable to the prolactin-inhibiting action of CB 154".

### (g) Teratology Studies in Rabbits

"CB 154 (micronized) was given to pregnant rabbits (yellow silver breed) at four dose levels—3, 10, 30 and 100 mg/kg/day—from days 6–18 *post coitum*. In a supplementary study, two additional doses—300 and 1000 mg/kg/day—were given to pregnant rabbits over the same time span. The purpose of these additional doses was to characterize the toxic effects of CB 154 on pregnant females, so that findings in the fetuses could be set in relation to maternal toxicity. The drug was administered in 2% gelatin by gavage, and controls received plain gelatin. The dams were sacrificed at term and examined together with their fetuses, maternal and fetal parameters being evaluated statistically.

"3 and 10 mg/kg/day were well tolerated by the dams. Doses of 30 mg/kg/day and above were subtoxic or toxic to the dams. At these doses, a questionable increase in prenatal mortality and in the incidence of fetal abnormalities was noted. These findings are considered to be the result of a toxic action of the drug on the dam, and it is concluded that CB 154 does not exert any embryolethal or teratogenic activity in the rabbit when given in non-toxic doses".

Although most Drug Regulatory Authorities agreed with the interpretation that the fetal anomalies which occurred in litters from mother rabbits receiving 30 mg/kg/day or more reflected general maternal toxicity rather than a specific embryotoxic or teratological action of bromocriptine, the U.S.A. authorities (FDA) were nevertheless concerned about the occurrence of three fetuses with cleft palates in the 100 mg/kg/day/group (one control fetus also exhibited this anomaly). As a result, they insisted that women of childbearing age should be instructed to use a mechanical form of contraception whilst under bromocriptine treatment. Repetition of the rabbit teratology study in another strain failed to reveal such anomalies, although two fetuses with cleft palates occurred in a repeat high-dose study in the original strain (see p. 43). Two teratology studies in monkeys subsequently showed that bromocriptine was not teratogenic in primates (see p. 44) and the results of more than 1400 documented pregnancies in women taking bromocriptine show that the drug is, indeed, without teratogenic effects in humans (see p. 54).

*(h) Fertility Study in Female Rats*

"Female rats were given CB 154 orally at doses of 1 and 3 mg/kg/day during the entire test period. Fourteen days after the start of medication, they were mated with untreated males. Half the females were killed 13 days *post coitum* and examined; the other half were allowed to deliver and rear their offspring until 21 days *post partum*, before being killed and examined together with their offspring.

"CB 154 was found to have no effects on the fertility of the dams, embryonic development or post natal viability of the offspring. The only noteworthy finding was a dose-dependent reduction of weight gain in the offspring during lactation, due to the expected inhibitory effect of CB 154 on lactation in the dams".

These reproduction studies demonstrated the absence of a teratogenic or embryotoxic effect of bromocriptine and showed that it did not affect fertility, embryonic development or post natal development in rats. With the exception of the 62 week dog study, all the studies mentioned in this section (i.e. "Extended Animal Toxicity Tests") were documented by August 1972. The British and U.S.A. Drug Regulatory Authorities granted permission to conduct clinical trials in the indication of lactation inhibition on the strength of this data in the Autumn of the same year. By this time the presence of prolactin in humans had been established (Frantz and Kleinberg 1970; Lewis *et al.*, 1971; Hwang *et al.*, 1972) and a radioimmunoassay developed (Hwang *et al.*, 1971). This made the task of assessing the ability of bromocriptine to inhibit prolactin secretion in humans considerably more objective and it was not long before the reduction of serum prolactin levels by bromocriptine in both puerperal women and patients with galactorrhoea was confirmed (Brun del Re *et al.*, 1973; Besser *et al.*, 1972).

In addition to the trials conducted in Britain and the U.S.A., clinical investigations were continued and extended in Europe. Based on results of the original fluorescence microscopy studies by Fuxe's Group in Stockholm which suggested that bromocriptine possesses central dopaminergic actions (Hökfelt and Fuxe, 1972), and additional neurochemical and behavioral studies which subsequently confirmed this (for review see Thorner *et al.*, 1980) it was decided to test bromocriptine in acromegaly and Parkinson's disease. The idea of testing bromocriptine in acromegaly stemmed from the observation that serum growth hormone (GH) falls in some acromegalics following levodopa administration (Liuzzi *et al.*, 1972). However, levodopa itself was far from being satisfactory, because of its short duration of action. The same group tried bromocriptine and found that a single oral dose of 2.5 mg reduced plasma GH for several hours in a group of acromegalic patients. The extent of the animal toxicity data available at that time was perfectly adequate to support the sort of long term clinical trial then necessary to establish the efficacy of bromocriptine in this new indication. These studies started in 1974 and by the following year it was clear that the clinical and metabolic responses to therapy were excellent (for review see Thorner *et al.*, 1980). Bromocriptine has now emerged as the first effective medical therapy for acromegaly.

Once the potent and selective central dopaminergic action of bromocriptine in animals had been established, treatment of Parkinson's disease became an obvious goal. Again the currently available animal toxicity data were adequate to support the long term clinical trials needed to confirm efficacy in this disease, even though it soon became clear that higher doses would be required to treat Parkinsonism (20–60 mg daily) than were required in hyperprolactinemia or acromegaly (5–15 mg daily). The first trials started in 1973 and the results were published the following year (Calne *et al.*, 1974a, b). Many clinical trials have been conducted since and bromocriptine is now confirmed as an effective anti-Parkinsonian agent which is useful in the management of some, but not all, patients (for review see Thorner *et al.*, 1980).

During the period 1972–1976 it became clear that disorders of prolactin secretion are not as uncommon as was originally believed. Since early trials had shown bromocriptine to be effective in restoring menstruation in women with amenorrhoea associated with galactorrhoea, it was also decided to investigate the usefulness of bromocriptine in the treatment of secondary amenorrhoea. Studies which were initially run in Britain, The Netherlands and France showed that therapy was successful (return of menstruation, ovulation, pregnancy) in over 90% of the cases where hyperprolactinemia was present and in 20–40% with normoprolactinemia (the latter is sometimes referred to as hypogonadism). The cases which responded to bromocriptine were characterized by an improvement in luteal function (Del Pozo *et al.*, 1976). Cases of hyperprolactinemia in men are commonly associated with impotence and diminished libido and here bromocriptine restored potency and increased testosterone levels (Franks *et al.*, 1978).

## 3. Registration Toxicity Studies

### (a) Background

In 1975 clinical trials for the use of bromocriptine as an inhibitor of lactation had been completed and the drug was registered and marketed in South Africa, Switzerland and Britain for this indication. At that time it was already obvious that bromocriptine was also going to be registered and marketed for secondary amenorrhoea, acromegaly and Parkinson's disease on a world-wide basis. Since some of these indications require long-term therapy, animal tests to investigate the carcinogenic potential of bromocriptine as well as additional reproduction studies were initiated. A series of mutagenicity tests were also performed. Nowadays the sequence of events for animal toxicity testing is somewhat different. At least one mutagenicity test, usually the Ames test using *Salmonella* bacteria, is routinely performed prior to the first administration of the compound to humans. However, mutagenicity tests were just beginning to be performed by the pharmaceutical industry then, so our procedure very much reflected the state of the art at that time. Today carcinogenicity tests in at least two species are required by most authorities before the compound can be registered. In some cases, depending on the chemical structure of the compound, its performance in mutagenicity tests and the duration of the trials required to demonstrate efficacy, such carcinogenicity tests are required even before long-term clinical testing can begin.

### (b) 100-Week oral Toxicity and Carcinogenicity Study in Rats

One control and three dose groups were given bromocriptine mixed in their food at concentrations which provided a mean daily drug intake of 1.8 mg/kg, 9.9 mg/kg and 44.5 mg/kg for 100 weeks. The observations made and the parameters measured were: mortality and clinical signs (daily), body weights, food intake, externally visible masses (weekly), full hematology, blood and urine chemistry and urinalysis (after weeks 6, 13, 26, 52, 78 and 99), ophthalmoscopy (weeks 52/53 and 99), full necropsy and histological work up of all major organ systems (ca. 40 organs/rat) immediately following the spontaneous death of the animal or at the termination of the study. Weights of major organs were also recorded. The results of the study are summarized in Table 1. The conclusions drawn from this study were as follows:

"The mid- and high-doses are clearly toxic. Almost all findings can be explained by the strong pharmacodynamic action (i.e. inhibition of prolactin release) of CB 154. The low dose can be regarded as a 'no-toxic-effect' level for CB 154 when given orally to rats for 2 years, based on the results of this study.

"CB 154 caused a significant, dose-dependent decrease in the overall number of tumors (controls 102, low dose 88, mid-dose 76, high-dose 48). This reflected a general decrease in the incidence of mammary tumors in females and adrenal tumors in males—both effects probably related to the prolactin inhibitory action of CB 154. Conversely CB 154 increased the incidence of uterine neoplasia at the mid- and high-dose levels. These CB 154-induced uterine neoplasms have been the subject of a series of additional experiments where it was shown that they result from an interaction between the drug's classical inhibitory effect on prolactin secretion and specific features of the waning endocrine system of the aging female rat. Thus these neoplasms have no relevance for man. A detailed documentation of these additional rat studies together with relevant human data, dated August 2nd, 1977, has already been made available to Drug Regulatory Authorities.

"Based on the results of the present study and on those included in the above-mentioned document, it can be concluded that CB 154 does not possess carcinogenic potential for man".

The additional experiments referred to in the above text are those which have already been discussed on pages 29–32. It was not unexpected that the hyperplastic and metaplastic lesions observed in the uteri of rats treated with bromocriptine for 53 weeks should progress to neoplasia when the duration of treatment was extended to 100 weeks. This is a simple manifestation of prolonged estrogen dominance brought about by the prolactin inhibitory effect of bromocriptine superimposed on the waning endocrine system of the aging female rat. It was clear to us at Sandoz, as well as to the Drug Regulatory Authorities and their scientific consultants, that these findings were not relevant for the human situation. Clinical experience has shown this interpretation to be correct.

The significant reductions in mammary tumors in females and adrenal tumors in males are interesting observations. A reduction in the frequency

TABLE 1. Results of a 100 week oral toxicity and carcinogenicity test in rats treated with bromocriptine

| | Controls (0) | | Low Dose (1.8 mg/kg/day) | | Mid Dose (9.9 mg/kg/day) | | High Dose (44.5 mg/kg/day) | |
|---|---|---|---|---|---|---|---|---|
| | Males 50 | Females 50 | Males 50 | Females 50 | Males 50 | Females 50 | Males 50 | Females 50 |
| Number of Rats | 50 | 50 | 50 | 50 | 50 | 50 | 50 | 50 |
| *Clinical Observations*[a] | | | | | | | | |
| Deaths | 36 | 32 | 28 | 25 | 21[c] | 23 | 19[d] | 32 |
| Reduced feed intake and body weight gain | — | — | slight | slight | slight | slight | slight | — |
| Excitability | — | — | — | slight | — | slight | — | slight |
| Serum triglycerides | — | — | — | → | → | → | → | → |
| Serum cholesterol | — | — | ← | — | → | → | → | → |
| Urinary Na$^+$ and K$^+$ | — | — | — | ← | ← | ← | ← | ← |
| Urinary Ca$^{2+}$ | — | — | — | → | — | ← | — | ← |
| *Post Mortem Observations*[a] | | | | | | | | |
| **(a) Non-Neoplastic Pathology** | | | | | | | | |
| Moderate/Severe Nephropathy | 42 | 8 | 31[b] | 4 | 31[b] | 0[c] | 21[d] | 0[c] |
| Polyarteritis Nodosa | 25 | 9 | 8[d] | 2[b] | 16[b] | 3 | 12[c] | 0[c] |
| Inflammatory, hyperplastic and metaplastic endometrial changes | — | 5 | — | 35[d] | — | 41[d] | — | 42[d] |
| Reduced luteal tissue in ovaries | — | — | — | +++ | — | +++ | — | +++ |
| **(b) Neoplastic Pathology** | | | | | | | | |
| Pituitary tumors | 4 | 7 | 2 | 8 | 0 | 3 | 3 | 1 |
| Thyroid tumors | 4 | 6 | 10 | 8 | 5 | 6 | 2 | 3 |
| Adrenal tumors | 19 | 2 | 12 | 2 | 14 | 1 | 3[c] | 1 |
| Pancreatic islet cell tumors | 2 | 0 | 1 | 0 | 3 | 1 | 3 | 0 |
| Testes tumors | 1 | — | 1 | — | 2 | — | 2 | — |
| Benign mammary tumors | — | 37 | — | 14[c] | — | 10[c] | — | 8[c] |
| Malignant mammary tumors | — | 3 | — | 1 | — | 0 | — | 0 |
| Benign uterine tumors | — | 0 | — | 0 | — | 1 | — | 0 |
| Malignant uterine tumors | — | 0 | — | 2 | — | 7[c] | — | 9[c] |
| Miscellaneous tumors | 12 | 3 | 16 | 7 | 15 | 4 | 10 | 3 |
| Total tumors | 42 | 58 | 42 | 42 | 39 | 33 | 23 | 25 |
| Tumor-bearing rats | 28 | 44 | 30 | 29[c] | 28 | 26[c] | 19 | 20[c] |

[a] Only parameters which were influenced by medication are listed. [b] P > 0.05; [c] P > 0.01; [d] P > 0.001 versus controls (Fishers Exact Test).

and malignancy of mammary tumors is a well known effect of prolactin suppression in rodents (Heuson *et al.*, 1970; Welsch and Gribler, 1973; Welsch and Nagasawa, 1977). Unfortunately this does not have particular relevance for man—only a small proportion of mammary tumors are prolactin-dependent in women, and such tumors often lose their hormonal dependence specificity during the course of treatment (Heuson *et al.*, 1972; Morgan *et al.*, 1976). The decreased numbers of adrenocortical tumors in male rats at the high dose level may also reflect chronic prolactin suppression, since prolactin can support the growth of such experimentally-induced tumors in rats, and may even, in fact, be involved in their induction (Thomson *et al.*, 1973). This observation may be relevant to the human situation because encouraging results have been obtained with bromocriptine in Cushing's disease (for review see Thorner *et al.* 1980).

Most of the other effects of long-term bromocriptine treatment which manifested themselves during the course of this study were also observed in the 53-week rat study and have been discussed already. However, the dramatic reduction in the incidence and severity of polyarteritis nodosa which occurred even at the lowest dose level is truly remarkable (see Fig. 3). Although this is an extremely common disease in laboratory rats, it occurs only rarely in man. Its etiology is uncertain, the most popular hypothesis being that it is autoimmune in nature (Wigley, 1970). The results of this long-term study suggest the possible involvement of prolactin in the etiology of this disease. Further investigations are currently being performed.

Overall this life time rat study did not reveal target-organ toxicity or carcinogenic effects of bromocriptine which are relevant for its clinical usage.

## (c) A Cancerogenic Potential Study in Mice

CB 154 was given mixed in the feed, to OF1 mice for 74 weeks. Four hundred mice were evenly divided into one control and three dose groups. The mean doses were 2, 10 and 50 mg/kg/day. The parameters measured and observations made were: mortality (daily), body weights, observation and palpation for external tumors and clinical signs (weekly), hematology (at the end of the study). Full necropsy was performed on all mice with histological work up of major organ systems. The results are summarized in Table 2.

"Body weight gain was dose-proportionally reduced in the female mice of the higher doses. At the beginning of the experiment dose-dependent pilo-erection and increased excitability were also seen in these doses. The high dose induced in addition a slight decrease of the leukocytes mean values.

"There was no evidence that tumors occurred more frequently or earlier, or were of a different type in the treated mice than in the controls. It is

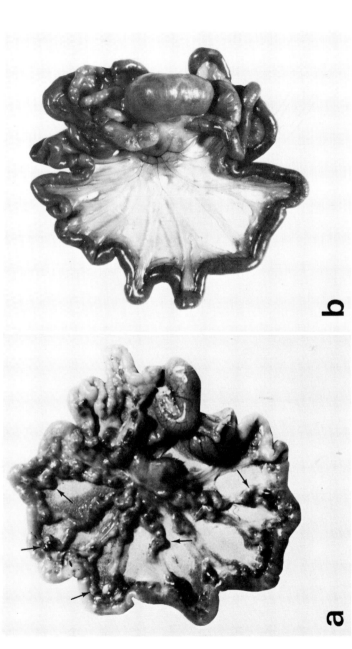

FIG. 3. Macroscopic appearance of the mesenteric vascular tree of male rats from a 100 week oral toxicity study. (a) Control rat with lesions typical of polyarteritis nodosa. The mesenteric arteries are massively dilated and tortuous and have many "pea-like" thickenings along their length (arrows). The lumina of these arteries show multiple aneurysms and thrombus formation. About 50% of control male rats were affected by this disease. (b) Rat treated with 1.8 mg/kg/day bromocriptine. The appearance of the mesenteric vessels is normal. Only 8% of treated rats had polyarteritis nodosa.

TABLE 2. Results of a 74 week oral carcinogenicity test in mice treated with bromocriptine

| | Controls (0) | | Low Dose (2 mg/kg/day) | | Mid Dose (10 mg/kg/day) | | High Dose (50 mg/kg/day) | |
|---|---|---|---|---|---|---|---|---|
| | Males | Females | Males | Females | Males | Females | Males | Females |
| Number of Mice | 50 | 50 | 50 | 50 | 50 | 50 | 50 | 50 |
| *Clinical Observations*[a] | | | | | | | | |
| Deaths | 24 | 23 | 18 | 16 | 26 | 17 | 32 | 21 |
| Piloerection | — | — | — | — | slight | — | slight | slight |
| Excitability | — | — | — | — | — | — | — | slight |
| Impaired body weight gain | — | — | — | — | — | + | — | ++ |
| Decreased leukocytes | — | — | — | — | slight | — | slight | slight |
| *Post Mortem Observations* | | | | | | | | |
| *Neoplastic Pathology* | | | | | | | | |
| Lung tumors | 19 | 10 | 15 | 11 | 10 | 11 | 17 | 7 |
| Lymphoreticular tumors | 15 | 22 | 8 | 16 | 14 | 18 | 14 | 22 |
| Liver tumors | 19 | 1 | 17 | 3 | 20 | 1 | 20 | 0 |
| Uterus/vagina tumors | — | 1 | — | 1 | — | 2 | — | 1 |
| Miscellaneous tumors | 2 | 6 | 1 | 2 | 0 | 5 | 3 | 5 |
| Total tumors | 55 | 40 | 41 | 33 | 44 | 37 | 54 | 35 |

[a]Only parameters which were influenced by medication are listed.

therefore concluded that CB 154 has no cancerogenic potential when given orally to mice".

There were no findings of interest made in this study other than the anticipated absence of a tumorigenic effect of bromocriptine on the uteri of treated mice.

### (d) Additional Teratology Studies in Rabbits

As previously mentioned, three fetuses with cleft palates were found in mother rabbits treated with 100 mg/kg/day. One such anomaly was also found in a control fetus. This was not considered relevant for the human situation because the mothers were given a dose which was clearly toxic. In a repeat study, identical in design except that the mother rabbits received 100 and 300 mg/kg/day from day 6 to day 18 post conception, this finding was reproduced—this time it occurred in two fetuses at the higher dose level only.

In a further study conducted with New Zealand white rabbits using an identical experimental protocol no cleft palates were produced. This suggests that the effects seen in yellow silver rabbits may be breed specific. Certainly they only occur at doses 100 times those used clinically and at ones which are clearly toxic to the mothers. When studies were conducted in both breeds to investigate the effects of bromocriptine on the pre-implantation phase of pregnancy (i.e. 100 or 300 mg/kg/day from day 1 to day 6 post conception), there was no evidence of an adverse effect on the onset of pregnancy or relevant changes in litter and fetal parameters. In New Zealand white rabbits some embryonic mortality occurred at the 300 mg/kg dose, which was again a reflection of overt maternal toxicity.

None of these studies revealed effects which were considered prohibitive for the use of bromocriptine in pregnant women.

### (e) Peri- and Postnatal Studies in Rats

"Female rats were treated with CB 154 (3, 10 and 30 mg/kg respectively) from day 15 *post coitum* until delivery. Post natal development of the offspring was followed up and behavior tests were performed. A limited number of pups were also investigated on reaching maturity with respect to fertility and pregnancy outcome.

"At the 3 and 10 mg/kg dose levels CB 154 was well tolerated by the dams, whereas at the 30 mg/kg dose level a reduced weight gain of the dams during treatment was found. Concerning the pregnancy outcome and the post natal development of the offspring, no marked changes occurred in the 3 and 10 mg/kg groups, whereas an increased pre- and perinatal as well as post natal mortality and a decreased weight gain of the pups was found in the 30 mg/kg group. This is explained by the impairment of lactation which is induced by the well-known inhibitory effect of CB 154 on prolactin secretion. Observation and testing of behavior revealed normal results in all dose groups.

"In view of the toxicity of the 30 mg/kg dose to the dams, these moderate changes are not of relevance and would not contraindicate clinical use of CB 154 in man".

### (f) A Fertility Study in Male Rats

"Male rats were treated orally with CB 154 (2, 10 and 50 mg/kg respectively). 70 days after the start of treatment they were paired with untreated virgin females. After mating, half of the females were killed on day 13 *post coitum* (p.c.) and examined; the other half were allowed to rear their young until day 21 *post partum* before being killed and examined together with their offspring.

"CB 154 was well tolerated in doses of 2 and 10 mg/kg. In the males treated with 50 mg/kg a distinctly reduced weight gain occurred. This dose group also showed the lowest copulation and fertility incidence, but was still within the normal range. As to the results obtained in the pregnant females, there was no remarkable finding in the subgroup examined on day 13 p.c. In the subgroup being allowed to deliver and rear the young, an increased pre- and perinatal mortality occurred in the 50 mg/kg group.

"In view of the toxicity of the 50 mg/kg dose, this moderate increase is not considered relevant. In the well tolerated dose range CB 154 had no adverse effect on the fertility of male rats or on the pre- and postnatal development of their offspring".

It is quite possible that, at the highest dose level employed, LH inhibition occurred in addition to prolactin inhibition and that this influenced both the fertility of the male rats and the viability of their offspring (Marko and Flückiger, 1973).

### (g) Total Reproductive Capacity in Female Mice

"CB 154 was given to female mice which were then tested for their total reproduction capacity. The orally administered single dose of 350 mg/kg had no negative effect on the fertility of the females during the one year experiment period. CB 154 can therefore be regarded as having no fertility-reducing effect on female germ cells, based on the results of this test".

### (h) Reproduction Studies in Stumptailed Monkeys

(i) *Teratology Study* "6 pregnant stumptailed macaques were treated orally with CB 154 at doses of 2 mg/kg/day, during organogenesis (between days 20 and 39 *post coitum*). The drug was given in gelatin capsules. The results were compared with those from 22 accumulated control pregnancies.

The drug was well tolerated and had no influence on the mothers or their fetuses. CB 154 had no embryolethal or teratogenic effect in the stumptailed macaque at the dose used".

*(ii) Effects on Menstrual Cycle, Fertility and Embryonic Development* "Fifteen female stumptailed macaques (*Macaca arctoides*) were treated orally with 0.15 mg/kg CB 154 twice daily for one or more cycles as well as for the subsequent pregnancy. In ten females, treatment was stopped on about day 30 *post coitum* (p.c.) while in the remaining five females it was terminated on the day of cesarean section (day 80 p.c.). The compound was mixed with molasses and given in rice paper sachets. The fetuses were delivered by cesarean section and examined.

"The drug was well tolerated by the dams, and no drug-related impairment of the body weight was observed. CB 154 had no influence on cycle length, ovulation, or conception. No malformations were found in the fetuses obtained. Three of the fifteen treated pregnancies ended in abortion, although signs of impending miscarriage were also observed in three of the ten control pregnancies. This finding is considered to be of no consequence as it is known that CB 154 does not cause a higher abortion rate in women than other substances used for the treatment of secondary amenorrhea. In the present study, CB 154 did not impair the fertility of female stumptailed macaques and was free of teratogenic effects as already seen in a previous teratological study in the same species".

*(i) Mutagenicity Studies*

*(i) Mutagenicity using Salmonella typhimurium* CB 154 was evaluated for mutagenic activity at concentrations ranging from 1 to 1000 $\mu$g/plate in *Salmonella typhimurium* strains TA 1535, TA 1538, with and without the addition of S9 fraction of liver homogenate obtained from female CD-1 mice. In a second study strains TA 1535, TA 1537, TA 1538, TA 98 and TA 100 were employed. Here concentrations of bromocriptine ranging from 3 to 3000 $\mu$g/plate were used with and without the addition of an S9 fraction of liver homogenate obtained from Aroclor-pretreated rats. Bromocriptine did not prove to be mutagenic under these conditions.

*(ii) Micronucleus test for Chromosome damaging Potential in Mice\** "In order to evaluate a possible mutagenic effect of CB 154, a micronucleus test was done using adult CD-1 mice. Each of five dose levels was given twice orally to four (or eight in the 400 mg/kg group) animals, the single doses

---

*Since pharmacokinetics were not performed in mice or Chinese hamsters (see p. 47), proof of the enteral absorbtion of bromocriptine in these species was previously established by conducting separate oral acute toxicity studies under conditions identical to those of the main study. The results were as follows: CD-1 mice: $LD_5$ 452 mg/kg, $LD_{50}$ 1269 mg/kg; Chinese hamsters: $LD_5$ 386 mg/kg, $LD_{50}$ 1269 mg/kg. Thus these mutagenicity studies were conducted with oral doses which were sufficiently large to achieve high plasma drug concentrations.

being 25, 100, 200, 400 or 600 mg/kg body weight. The mean percentages of micronucleated erythrocytes in bone marrow in control, 25, 100, 200, 400 and 600 mg/kg groups were 0.22, 0.10, 0.18, 0.20, 0.14 and 0.13, respectively, all of which were within normal limits (0.0–0.3%).

"CB 154 did not prove itself mutagenic in this test system".

*(iii) Cytogenetic Analysis of Chinese Hamster Bone Marrow Cells for Evaluation of Chromosome damaging Potential** "In order to evaluate a possible mutagenic effect of CB 154, a chromosome examination and micronucleus test of bone marrow cells were done using Chinese hamsters. Each of two dose-levels was given twice orally with an interval of 24 h to six animals in the chromosome test, the single doses being 100 and 400 mg/kg body weight. Each of three dose-levels was given orally with an interval of 24 h to four animals in the micronucleus test, the single doses being 25, 100 and 400 mg/kg body weight. The mean percentages of metaphases with chromosome aberrations in control, 100 mg/kg and 400 mg/kg groups were 1.67, 1.00 and 0.67, respectively, all of which were within control limits (0.0–2.0%).

"The mean percentages of micronucleated erythrocytes in the bone marrow in control, 25 mg/kg, 100 mg/kg and 400 mg/kg groups amounted to 0.13, 0.20, 0.30 and 0.28, respectively. These values were within normal limits (0.0–0.3%). CB 154 did not prove itself mutagenic in these two test systems".

*(iv) Dominant Lethal Test in Male Mice for Evaluation of Chromosome damaging Potential in Germ Cells** "CB 154 was tested for dominant lethal activity in male CD-1 mice. No mutagenic effects on any stage of spermatogenesis were detected when the drug was administered orally by stomach tube, single-dose administration, at concentrations up to 300 mg/kg body weight. There was no antifertility effect of CB 154 on the treated males as shown by the frequency of successful mating. There was no evidence of pre-implantation losses as indicated by the number of total implants per pregnant female. There was no evidence of significant post-implantation losses as shown by the number of dead and living implants per pregnancy, which were all within normal limits".

4. Conclusions from Animal Toxicity Data

The extremely comprehensive and detailed series of animal toxicity tests described above (see also Table 3), which required almost ten years to complete, finally permitted the conclusion that bromocriptine is not teratogenic, embryotoxic, mutagenic or carcinogenic and does not possess the potential to induce target organ toxicity in animals. The effects associated with the long-term administration of very high doses reflected

*See footnote on p. 45.

exaggerated pharmacodynamic actions of the compound (inhibition of prolactin secretion or central dopaminergic effects), or were non-specific in nature. As the next section shows, clinical experience subsequently confirmed that these conclusions were valid for the use of bromocriptine in humans.

This data has permitted the registration and marketing of bromocriptine for the treatment of prolactin secreting pituitary adenomas, acromegaly, post partum and post abortion lactation, post partum mammary congestion, incipient puerperal mastitis, galactorrhoea with or without amenorrhoea, prolactin-dependent premenstrual symptoms, prolactin-dependent menstrual disorders and subfertility, prolactin-dependent male hypogonadism, impotence and oligospermia and Parkinsonism in more than 100 countries.


## IV. Pharmacokinetics and metabolism in animals and man

### A. Pharmacokinetic Studies in the Rat, Rabbit, Rhesus Monkey and Man Using $^3$H-Bromocriptine

"Absorption, blood levels and urinary and fecal excretion of the radioactivity were studied in the rat, rabbit and monkey following single oral and intravenous administration. In man absorption, blood levels and urinary excretion were measured after single oral and intravenous administration. Fecal excretion was determined in a separate bioavailability study with $^{14}$C-CB 154. In addition the biliary excretion was studied in rat and rhesus monkey. The distribution of radioactivity throughout the body was determined in rat.

"The results of the study can be summarized as follows. Low blood concentrations, a small urinary excretion and a high biliary excretion are the main features of the pharmacokinetics in all species investigated. The absorption of the drug after oral administration is fairly good and amounts to about 40–90% in rat, rabbit and monkey. In man even higher values were calculated. The absorption was determined from renal excretion data in rat, rhesus monkey and man, from blood levels in the rat, rabbit and rhesus monkey, and finally from biliary and urinary excretion data of rats and rhesus monkeys with bile duct fistula.

"The percentages of drug absorbed calculated from blood level integrals and from renal excretion data are rather inaccurate values due to the low blood levels, their inaccurate extrapolation to infinite times and the small ratio of the dose excreted into urine independent of the route of administration. Since the bile is the main route of excretion, the most reliable data for absorption are obtained from animals with a bile duct fistula.

TABLE 3. Overview of the animal toxicity tests performed with bromocriptine from 1968–1979

| Type of Study | Species | No. Animals per Group | Dosage Schedule | Duration of Drug Administration[a] | Examinations[b] | Date of Completion |
|---|---|---|---|---|---|---|
| **1. PRECLINICAL TOXICITY STUDIES** | | | | | | |
| Acute toxicity | Rat | 10 ♂/♀ } | Single intravenous and oral dose | 14 days observation | Signs of acute overdosage; LD$_{50}$ values | March 1968 |
| | Rabbit | 6 ♂/♀ } | | | | |
| | Mouse | 10 ♂/♀ | | | | |
| Subacute oral toxicity | Rat | 5 ♂, 5 ♀ | 10, 30, 100 mg/kg/day in feed | 4 weeks | Routine Set* | June 1968 |
| | Dog | 1 ♂, 1 ♀ | 1, 4, 16 mg/kg/day orally in gelatin capsules | 4 weeks | | May 1968 |
| Teratology study | Rat | 25 ♀ | 3, 10, 30 mg/kg/day by stomach tube suspended in 2% gelatin | days 6–15 p.c. | Routine Set** | Feb. 1979 |
| **2. EXTENDED TOXICITY TESTS** | | | | | | |
| Chronic oral toxicity | Rat | 15 ♂, 15 ♀ | 5, 20, 82 mg/kg/day in feed | 53 weeks | Routine Set** | March 1972 |
| | Rat | 15 ♂, 15 ♀ | 19 mg/kg/day in feed | 13 weeks | | March 1972 |
| | Dog | 3 ♂, 3 ♀ | 1, 3, 10 mg/kg/day oral in gelatin capsules | 62 weeks | | April 1973 |
| | Rhesus monkey | 2 ♂, 2 ♀ | 2, 8, 32 mg/kg/day by stomach tube in 0.5% Tragacanth | 13 weeks | | July 1972 |
| Teratology studies | Rat | 10 ♀ } | 3, 10, 30 mg/kg/day by stomach tube suspended in 2% gelatin | days 6–15 p.c. | | July 1972 |
| | Rat | 30 ♀ } | | days 8–15 p.c. | Routine Set** | July 1972 |
| | Rabbit | 17 ♀ | 3, 10, 30, 100 mg/kg/day by stomach tube in 2% gelatin | days 6–18 p.c. | | July 1972 |
| | | 5 ♀ | 300, 1000 mg/kg/day by stomach tube in 2% gelatin | days 6–18 p.c. | | July 1972 |
| Fertility study | Rat | 15 ♀ | 1, 3 mg/kg/day by stomach tube in 2% gelatin | 15 days prior to mating—day 13 p.c. | Routine Set** | April 1972 |
| | | 15 ♀ | | 15 days prior to mating—day 21 p.p. | Routine set** + peri and postnatal mortality and body weight development of pups. | April 1972 |
| **3. REGISTRATION TOXICITY STUDIES** | | | | | | |
| Chronic toxicity and carcinogenicity study | Rats | 50 ♂, 50 ♀ | 1.8, 9.9, 44.5 mg/kg/day in feed | 100 weeks | Routine Set* | Oct. 1977 |
| Carcinogenicity study | Mice | 50 ♂, 50 ♀ | 2, 10, 50 mg/kg/day in feed | 74 weeks | Clinical signs, hematology, full necropsy and histology of all major organ systems | Sept. 1977 |

| Study | Species | No. | Dose | Parameters[b] | Treatment[a] | Date |
|---|---|---|---|---|---|---|
|  | (yellow silver) |  | tube in 2% gelatin |  |  | April 1976 |
|  | Rabbits (New Zealand Whites) | 15 ♀ | 100, 300 mg/kg/day stomach tube in 2% gelatin | Routine Set** | days 6–18 p.c. | April 1976 |
|  | Rabbits (yellow silver) | 15 ♀ | 100, 300 mg/kg/day by stomach tube in 2% gelatin | Routine Set** | days 1–6 p.c. | April 1976 |
|  | Rabbit (New Zealand Whites) | 15 ♀ | 100, 300 mg/kg/day by stomach tube in 2% gelatin | Routine Set** | days 1–6 p.c. | April 1976 |
|  | Monkeys (Maccaca arctoides) | 6 ♀ | 2 mg/kg/day orally in gelatin capsules | Food intake and clinical signs in mothers, fetal morphology, placental weights and appearance | days 20–39 p.c. | March 1976 |
| Peri- and postnatal development | Rats | 25 ♀ | 3, 10, 30 mg/kg/day by stomach tube in 2% gelatin | Routine Set** + behavioral tests on $F_1$ generation. Fertility of $F_1$ generation, fetal development of $F_2$ | days 15–20 p.c. and on day 0, 4, 21 p.p. | April 1976 |
| Fertility studies | Rats | 15 ♂ | 2, 10, 50 mg/kg/day by stomach tube in 2% gelatin | Routine Set** + Necropsy of treated males | 10 weeks before mating with untreated females | April 1976 |
| Fertility and embryonic development | Monkeys (Maccaca arctoides) | 15 ♀ | 0.15 mg/kg/2 × daily in rice paper sachets | Ovulation, fertility, course of pregnancy, fetal morphology | day prior to mating; till day 30 p.c. in 10 ♀, till day 80 p.c. in 5 ♀ | Dec. 1979 |
| Mutagenicity studies —Ames test | Salmonella bacteria | — | 1, 10, 100, 1000 µg/culture plate | Total number of colonies, number of revertant colonies | 48 hours | Jan. 1978 |
| Micronucleus test | Mice | 4–8 ♂/♀ | 25, 100, 200, 400, 600 mg/kg by stomach tube in 2% gelatin | Micronucleated erythrocytes in bone marrow | 2 administrations 24 h apart | March 1976 |
| Cytogenetic analysis of bone marrow | Chinese Hamster | 4 ♂/♀ | 25, 100, 400 mg/kg by stomach tube in 2% gelatin | Chromosome analysis and presence of micronucleated erythrocytes | 2 administrations 24 h apart |  |
|  |  | 6 ♂/♀ | 100, 400 mg/kg by stomach tube in 2% gelatin |  | 2 administrations 24 h apart | Sept. 1976 |
| Dominant lethal test | Mice | 40 ♂ | 100, 300 mg/kg by stomach tube in 2% gelatin | Pre or post implantation loss in untreated ♀, mated with treated ♂, fertility of ♂ | 1 administration | Jan. 1978 |
| Total reproductive capacity | Mice | 49 ♀ | 350 mg/kg by stomach tube in 2% gelatin | Number of litters and offspring produced in 1 year | 1 administration before being kept with male | Feb. 1979 |

[a] p.c. = post coitum; p.p. = post partum. [b] Routine Set* = Body weights, food intake, clinical signs, serum and urine chemistry, urinalysis, eye examinations, hematology, necropsy, organ weights, histology of all major organ systems. In dogs and monkeys, electrocardiography in addition. Routine Set** = Clinical signs in dams, pregnancy rate, body weights of dams, necropsy of dams, implantations, living fetuses/dam; prenatal mortality, fetal body weights, sex distribution of fetuses, fetal morphology, placental weights.

"The blood levels in all species are very similar. They are lower in oral experiments than after intravenous administration. Very low levels persisted for 4 days after oral administration.

"The organ levels (in rat) after i.v. or p.o. administration are low in the gastrointestinal tract and the liver and very low in other organs after 24 h.

"The recoveries of the radioactivity excreted are very satisfactory, indicating that there is no irreversible retention of the drug in the organism.

"The comparison of the data from man and the other species shows that the absorption determined in man by using the ratio:

$$\frac{\text{amount excreted into urine after p.o. administration}}{\text{amount excreted into urine after i.v. administration}}$$

results in $0.95 \pm 0.12$, which is even higher than the figures obtained for rat and monkey by the same method. Peak blood levels ($F = 0.14 \pm 0.04$ in man) and the shape of the blood level curves in man and animal are quite similar.

"The cumulative excretion of $^3$H-labeled material in the urine ($6.4 \pm 0.7\%$ of the dose after oral administration and $6.7 \pm 0.6\%$ after intravenous administration in man) are similar except for the rat which shows even lower values. The main part of the dose is excreted in all animal species via bile into feces.

. "For studies in man no patient with a cannulated bile duct has been used. But taking into account the great similarity of the biliary excretion in rat and monkey it can be assumed to be of the same order of magnitude in man".

## B. Metabolism studies in the rat, rhesus monkey and man

The metabolic fate of CB 154 has been studied using $^{14}$C-bromocriptine in rat, rhesus monkey and in man.

Only small traces of parent drug were found in the urine of the three species. The main metabolites in urine were identified as 2-bromo-lysergic acid and 2-bromo-isolysergic acid. The metabolic pattern is less complex in man than in rat and rhesus monkey.

No parent drug was found in the bile of rat and rhesus monkey. The metabolic pattern in the bile of both animal species is fairly complex, 27 distinct radioactive zones being localized by column and thin-layer chromatography.

Ten metabolites were isolated and their structures partially or completely elucidated. Twenty-nine metabolites in bile and urine were characterized by their elution volume, Rf-values and fluorescence. It has been proven that the positions 12, 13, and the 6-methyl group are not attacked to a major degree by the oxidative enzymes in the body. Three processes are going on in the body:

(1) isomerization at carbon atom 8 of the bromolysergic acid moiety,
(2) hydrolysis of the lysergic acid amine group (a minor pathway),
(3) oxidative attack on the proline fragment of the peptide moiety.

## V. Human clinical aspects

Bromocriptine was first marketed in 1975, for the suppression of post partum and post abortion lactation and for the treatment of prolactin-dependent menstrual disorders and subfertility. Subsequently it was used to treat prolactin secreting pituitary adenomas, acromegaly, post partum mammary congestion, incipient puerperal mastitis, galactorrhea with or without amenorrhoea, prolactin-dependent premenstrual symptoms, prolactin-dependent male hypogonadism impotence and oligospermia and Parkinsonism.

Several million patients have received bromocriptine since its introduction. Many of these have received long-term therapy, particularly those patients with acromegaly or Parkinson's disease.

In most hyperprolactinemic conditions low doses (2.5 mg to 7.5 mg daily) are sufficient for successful treatment. For patients with prolactinomas, higher doses (up to 20 mg daily) may be required for adequate control of serum prolactin levels. In acromegaly an average dose of 15 mg daily appears to be necessary to maintain continuous suppression of growth hormone secretion. The highest doses are used in Parkinsonian patients; on average 30 mg daily are required; however, doses up to 150 mg have been used (Calne, 1978).

## A. Adverse Reactions

### 1. Generally

Side effects have not been a major problem. Several million patients have received bromocriptine and, as would be expected in any population as large as this, many of whom suffer from serious diseases, fatalities have occurred concomitantly with bromocriptine therapy. To date there is no evidence that bromocriptine was the responsible factor in any of these cases.

Non-fatal, minor and major adverse reactions have produced a wide range of symptoms; some are dependent on the disease for which the patient is being treated, the dosage of bromocriptine given, and the duration of treatment. The most frequently observed are nausea, vomiting and headache, all of which probably result from stimulation of central dopamine receptors. Postural hypotension, which can on rare occasions lead to collapse in sensitive patients, and gastrointestinal side effects such as abdominal pain, diarrhoea and constipation have also been reported. All these adverse effects may be minimized or even prevented by giving small initial doses of bromocriptine which are taken with a meal.

An untoward effect of minor importance is nasal stuffiness, the pharmacological mechanism of which is not clear but may involve $\alpha$-adrenoceptor or serotonin receptor interaction. These adverse reactions have been noticed in all kinds of patient and appear to be independent of the disease for which they are being treated. They appear to result from the pharmacodynamic properties of bromocriptine. In contrast, the adverse reactions discussed below show a clear dependence on the disease for which the patient is being treated.

## 2. Acromegalic patients

There have been occasional reports of gastro-intestinal bleeding, sometimes severe, in acromegalic patients receiving bromocriptine. Since this gastrointestinal bleeding has also been observed in untreated acromegalics or in those receiving alternative therapy, it is unlikely that bromocriptine is responsible. Actually, an increased occurrence of peptic ulcer is known to occur with acromegaly, and the frequency of gastro-intestinal bleeding in bromocriptine treated acromegalic patients is no higher than would be expected in an untreated population of acromegalics (Wass *et al.*, 1976b; Del Pozo and Maclay, 1976; Besser and Wass, 1978). Nevertheless, physicians are presently advised to give alternative treatment to acromegalic patients with a history or evidence of peptic ulceration. If bromocriptine has to be used in such patients, they should be instructed to report any gastro-intestinal reactions promptly.

Digital vasospasms, especially following exposure to cold, have been observed in some acromegalic patients who were on high dose regimes and who suffered previously from Raynaud's disease. Although bromocriptine is only a weak $\alpha$-adrenoceptor and serotonin receptor stimulating agent, this adverse effect may result from stimulation of such vascular receptors. After dose reduction these, usually minor, vascular disturbances disappear (Wass *et al.*, 1976a). Very occasionally digital vasospasm also occurs in patients treated with bromocriptine for diseases other than acromegaly (Duvoisin *et al.*, 1979). True ergotism has, however, never been observed with bromocriptine.

## 3. Parkinson's disease patients

Dopamine receptor agonists including bromo criptine can induce untoward psychic or neurological reactions. These untoward reactions have been noticed almost exclusively in Parkinsonian patients who had previously received L-DOPA. The symptoms include primarily visual hallucinations which are often brightly colored. Auditory hallucinations are uncommon. Confusion, delusions and psychomotor excitation have also been noticed (Calne *et al.*, 1978). Predisposed to these symptoms are elderly patients who have already been on anti-Parkinson drugs for long periods prior to receiving bromo criptine or who receive, in addition to bromocriptine, other centrally acting drugs. On the other hand, results of animal studies showing bromocriptine to possess antidepressant properties have been confirmed by clinical studies (Theohar *et al.*, 1981).

Involuntary movements including dyskinesia are the main neurological adverse reaction of bromocriptine treatment in Parkinson's disease. The etiology and pathogenesis of this side effect is poorly understood. However the dyskinesias are similar to those seen in patients receiving L-DOPA; they tend to become more prominent as the disease progresses (March, 1979). Involuntary movements have never been observed in patients taking bromocriptine for other indications, e.g. hyperprolactinemic conditions or acromegaly.

Rarely erythromelalgia—warm, red and swollen ankles—may develop in Parkinsonian patients receiving relatively high doses of bromocriptine. These symptoms gradually regress if the dose is reduced (Calne *et al.*, 1978; Calne, 1978).

When pleuropulmonary changes of undetermined etiology, in particular pleural effusions, were recently reported in some Parkinsonian patients on long-term therapy at one Finnish clinic (Rinne, 1981), two surveys were performed. These showed that in 779 Parkinsonian patients such changes occurred with the same frequency in bromocriptine and non-bromocriptine-treated Parkinsonian patients (Krupp, 1981 and unpublished data). However, although exudative or fibrotic lung reactions have never been observed in other long-term studies, the possibility of an association between exudative–fibrotic pleuropulmonary changes and bromocriptine therapy could not be entirely excluded. It is now recommended that Parkinsonian patients on long-term bromocriptine therapy who present unexplained signs or symptoms of pleuropulmonary dysfunction be examined thoroughly and discontinuation of bromocriptine considered.

## 4. Acute overdosage

A few observations after acute overdosage in children and adults have been reported. No life threatening reactions have occurred. In all cases the most prominent symptom was nausea and vomiting. Patients taking up to 25 mg of bromocriptine for the first time may experience dizziness, hypotension and sweating.

# B. Drug interactions

No serious interactions with bromocriptine are known. It has, however, been reported that the frequency and intensity of adverse reactions to bromocriptine may be increased by the intake of alcohol (Ayres and Maisey, 1980), and similarly bromocriptine may decrease alcohol tolerance (Besser and Wass, 1979; Pelkonen *et al.*, 1980). The pathogenetic mechanism of this interaction has not been elucidated.

On theoretical grounds interactions between bromocriptine and various other drugs are potentially possible; for instance bromocriptine antagonizes the stimulatory effect of neuroleptics, tricyclic antidepressants, Rauwolfia alkaloids and estrogens on prolactin secretion in a dose-dependent manner (Flückiger *et al.*, 1982).

# C. Bromocriptine in pregnancy

When it became apparent that previously infertile women suffering from various hyperprolactinemic conditions may conceive while being treated with bromocriptine, a survey of the course and the outcome of these pregnancies was initiated. In 1973 clinicians who prescribed bromocriptine to women with endocrinological disorders were contacted. They were advised to inform their patients that this treatment may restore fertility and that they should use a mechanical form of contraception, unless they wish to conceive. It was recommended to stop medication as soon as pregnancy was confirmed. Since there is a delay between conception and confirmation of pregnancy, knowledge of the effects of bromocriptine treatment on early fetal development is extremely important. Clinicians were therefore asked to monitor patients carefully and to report on the course and outcome of each pregnancy. To date, detailed information is available on the outcome of more than 1400 pregnancies in women who were taking bromocriptine at the time of conception. A comparison with published control data suggests that bromocriptine treatment during pregnancy is associated neither with an adverse effect on its course nor with increased risk of spontaneous abortions, multiple pregnancies or congenital malformations. In particular there was no increase in the occurrence of babies with cleft palates. Moreover, a special investigation revealed that, in children born to mothers treated with bromocriptine during early pregnancy, no numerical or structural chromosomal anomalies occurred which could be ascribed to therapy (Schellekens *et al.*, 1977).

Preliminary results from a special and still on-going investigation do not indicate any adverse effects on the postnatal development of babies born to bromocriptine-treated mothers either.

In spite of these very reassuring results, a prospective large-scale intensive project is in progress at 35 leading hospitals in 12 countries in order to monitor the outcome of pregnancies resulting from and continuing under bromocriptine treatment. This is necessary to counter-balance the negative selection which obviously occurs when only spontaneous reporting of adverse outcomes occurs, and where no control group is available. Interim results from this project are very encouraging.

It has long been known that pituitary tumors of the chromophobe type increase in size during pregnancy and can cause complications (Child *et al.*, 1975). A survey, which by its very nature had to be limited to a small number of patients (116 completed pregnancies) revealed that only two of the women with pituitary tumors who were treated with bromocriptine suffered from complications necessitating surgical intervention during pregnancy (Griffith *et al.*, 1979). Nevertheless, careful supervision throughout pregnancy is essential if pregnancy occurs in a woman with a pituitary tumor. The precautionary measures include regular checking of the visual field.

## D. Gynecological Surveys

Although the uterine changes observed in rats treated for long periods with bromocriptine were considered to be a phenomenon peculiar to this species, their true relevance for humans could be accurately assessed only in the light of clinical experience. Two surveys which included gynecological and endometrial examination of patients treated for long periods of time with relatively high doses of bromocriptine, as well as circumstantial evidence from pregnancy surveys and reviews of all published data, provide no indication whatever that the drug induces uterine abnormalities (Besser *et al.*, 1977 and data from Sandoz Drug Monitoring Centre records).

## VI. Conclusions

The toxicological development of bromocriptine described in this chapter and summarized in Table 3 provides the reader with a good example of what is currently required before a new single chemical entity can be tested in man and subsequently registered and marketed as an ethical pharmaceutical speciality. The animal studies took over ten years to complete at a cost (1982 values) of 2.7 million Swiss francs. In rabbit teratology studies cleft palates occurred in a few fetuses from mothers given very high doses of bromocriptine, whilst in the long term rat study uterine tumors developed. These problems certainly put the further development of bromocriptine in jeopardy and only after extensive investigation could it be shown that neither of these effects was relevant for the use of the compound in humans. Of course, only subsequent clinical experience could provide the ultimate proof of bromocriptine's safety in man, and rigorous monitoring of all side effects was thus required throughout the various developmental phases. This continues even though the compound is now marketed, taking the form of so-called "Post Marketing Surveillance". As with all marketed compounds, our Drug Monitoring Centre is responsible for documenting and investigating all side effects which are reported to them as well as for performing the types of worldwide epidemiological studies referred to on p. 55, and which are required to answer questions specific to any special circumstances pertinent to the drug's use.

Do the benefits gained in terms of therapeutic and scientific progress justify the tremendous expenditure of time, effort, animal life and financial resources? There can be little doubt that they do in the case of bromocriptine. It is the first directly acting, selective dopamine receptor agonist. As such it provides the first effective medical treatment for prolactin-secreting pituitary tumors and acromegaly. In addition it represents a great improvement over existing therapy for the inhibition of physiological and pathological lactation, as well as for the treatment of certain kinds of male and female infertility, amenorrhoea and Parkinson's disease. Its potential usefulness in a series of further important indications is currently being assessed. The compound has also contributed significantly to the physiological, pharmacological and biochemical sciences, since it was the first potent and selective dopamine agonist and has therefore often been used as a tool to probe mechanisms of biological control at the cellular level. The knowledge gained from such experiments will undoubtedly result in the development of new and better drugs for many indications.

Thus we firmly believe that the benefit to patients and the scientific progress made with bromocriptine justify the investment with one reservation—the number of animal toxicity studies performed and the number of animals included in some of these were, in our opinion, excessive. They were nevertheless required to satisfy the differing demands of various drug regulatory bodies at that time. For instance it can be questioned whether it was really necessary to repeat the rabbit teratology studies when fetuses with cleft palates were only observed in litters born to mother rabbits which had previously received clearly toxic doses of bromocriptine.*

It could also be argued that the mutagenicity studies with bromocriptine

*On the other hand it must be remembered that one of the major clinical indications for bromocriptine is female infertility and the chances of drug therapy continuing during the organogenetic phase of early pregnancy are therefore high. Obviously, particular importance was placed on the results of the first rabbit teratology experiments by certain authorities in this case.

were excessive. However at the time they were performed the pharmaceutical industry was anticipating clear-cut guidelines from the various drug regulatory authorities on mutagenicity testing but did not know what these requirements would involve. Moreover the state of the science was such that it was not known that the results of the micronucleus test in mice and the cytogenetic analysis of bone marrow in hamsters correlate almost perfectly, making one of these tests unnecessary. In addition it is now appreciated that the total reproductive capacity test conducted after the administration of a single large dose of a compound to female mice is more likely to demonstrate a cytostatic action than a mutagenic one. In fact we no longer perform this test in our laboratories, since it is not considered to be critical for mutagenicity evaluation.

Finally we want to emphasize that bromocriptine was the first dopaminergic/prolactin secretion inhibiting compound that underwent a full toxicological development. Follow up compounds with a similar pharmacological profile will obviously benefit from the experience we have gained with bromocriptine, making fewer toxicological studies necessary for the clinical testing, registration and marketing of such analogues. Nevertheless the total reduction will not exceed 10–20%.

One cardinal question remains to be answered concerning the usefulness of animal tests: How accurate were they in predicting the side effects which were subsequently observed in man?* From animal pharmacological studies bromocriptine was characterized as a potent and selective dopaminergic agonist. Thus it was anticipated that it might cause vomiting, hallucinations, arterial hypotension and possibly dyskinesia in man. In addition, based on structural and pharmacological considerations (many ergot compounds are known to cause $\alpha$-adrenoreceptor blockade) one had to assume that bromocriptine might induce nasal stuffiness.

In contrast to the pharmacology studies, the predictive value of the animal toxicity studies may, at first, appear rather low (see Table 4). Nevertheless some human side effects were predicted. For instance salivation and vomiting which occurred in a dose-dependent manner in bromocriptine-treated dogs, reflect the nausea and vomiting which occur in man. Similarly impaired

---

*For those readers who are not themselves actively engaged in drug development it must be pointed out that what is *not* seen in animal studies is as important as what is, since the absence of major toxicity problems in animals is a prerequisite for the clinical testing, development, registration and marketing of a new drug. Remember that from our animal toxicity studies we predicted that bromocriptine would not cause serious toxicity problems such as fatal acute cardiovascular or central nervous phenomena, target organ toxicity, teratological effects, embryotoxic effects, damage to genetic material or cancer in man, and, according to current clinical experience, the prediction appears to have been reliable in each case. Thus the term "side effect", as used here, refers to the reversible and essentially minor symptoms that are usually associated with exaggerated pharmacodynamic actions of the compound in man.

TABLE 4. Comparison of untoward effects in animals and man

| Symptoms | Animal Toxicology Studies | Adverse Reactions in Man | Predicted from Pharmacology Properties |
|---|---|---|---|
| *CNS Effects* | | | |
| Hallucinations | — | (+) | + |
| Headache | — | + | — |
| Dyskinesia | — | (+) | + |
| Nausea | + (Dogs) | + | — |
| Salivation | + (Dogs) | — | — |
| Vomiting | + (Dogs) | + | + |
| *Cardiovascular Effects* | | | |
| Nasal Stuffiness | — | + | + |
| Orthostatic hypotension | — | + | — |
| Hypotension, arterial | — | + | + |
| Vasomotor reactions | + (Dogs) | (+) | — |
| *Gastro-intestinal Effects* | | | |
| Constipation | — | + | — |
| Peptic ulcer | — | (+)[c] | — |
| *Effects on Skin Appendages* | | | |
| Impaired hair growth | + (Rats, dogs) | +[a] | — |
| *Effects on Female Reproductive System* | | | |
| Uterine tumors | + (Rats) | — | — |
| *Effect on Reproduction* | | | |
| Teratogenicity | —[b] | — | — |
| Behavioral alterations in $F_1$ generation | — | — | — |
| *Effects on Respiratory System* | | | |
| Pleuropulmonary exudation/fibrosis | — | (+)[c] | — |

(+) Adverse reaction seen mainly or exclusively in one indication.
[a] Observed only rarely. [b] Occasional rabbit fetuses with cleft palates only occurred in litters of dams treated with such high doses of bromocriptine that the mother animals showed overt signs of toxicity; in view of this maternal toxicity, these studies were not considered to demonstrate a specific teratogenic action of bromocriptine. [c] A definite association with bromocriptine administration not yet established.

hair growth which was observed in rats and dogs given toxic or subtoxic doses of bromocriptine can also be seen on rare occasions in man; this side effect is reversible after discontinuing the drug in both animals and man. It should also be remembered that the animal studies accurately predicted that major toxicity problems would not occur in humans. Viewed in this light, the animal toxicity studies conducted with bromocriptine were indeed highly predictive of the situation in man.

Finally we should like to mention a positive aspect of animal toxicity studies which is generally overlooked. Since pharmacological studies are usually acute or subacute in nature, the chronic toxicity studies often provide the only opportunity to evaluate the possible beneficial aspects of long term drug administration in animals. Thus in our studies bromocriptine prevented the development of chronic renal disease, polyarteritis nodosa, adrenal cortical adenomas and mammary tumors in rats. Each of these observations has initiated clinical activity which may well lead to the identification of new indications for bromocriptine in the future.

# References

Ayres, J. and Maisey, M. N. (1980). Alcohol increases bromocriptine's side effects. *New Engl. J. Med.* **302**, 806.

Besser, G. M. and Wass, J. A. H. (1978). Medical management of acromegaly with bromocriptine: Effects of continuous treatment for over three years. *Med. J. Aust.* **2**, No. 3 (Spec. Suppl.), 31–33.

Besser, G. M., Parke, L., Edwards, C. R. W., Forsyth, I. A. and McNeilly, A. (1972). Galactorrhoea: successful treatment with reduction of plasma prolactin levels by brom-ergocryptine. *Br. med. J.* **3**, 669–672.

Besser, G. M., Thorner, M. O., Wass, J. A. H., Doniach, I., Canti, G., Curling, M., Grudziniskas, J. G. and Setchell, M. E. (1977). Absence of uterine neoplasia in patients on bromocriptine. *Br. med. J.* **2**, 868.

Brun, Del Re, R., Del Pozo, E., De Grandi, P., Friesen, H., Hinselmann, M. and Wyss, H. (1973). Prolactin inhibition and suppression of puerperal lactation by α-Br-ergocryptine (CB-154). A comparison with estrogen. *Obstet. Gynecol.* **41**, 884–890.

Calne, D. B. (1978). Bromocriptine and the nigrostriatal system: Parkinsonism. *Triangle (Biling.)* **17**, No. 1, 49–53.

Calne, D. B., Teychenne, P. F., Claveria, L. E., Eastman, R., Greenacre, J. K. and Petrie, A. (1974a). Bromocriptine in Parkinsonism. *Br. med. J.* **4**, 442.

Calne, D. B., Teychenne, P. F., Leigh, P. N., Bamji, A. N. and Greenacre, J. K. (1974b). Treatment of Parkinsonism with Bromocriptine. *Lancet*, **II**, 1355–1356.

Calne, D. B., Williams, A. D., Nutt, H. G., Neophytides, A., Eisler, T. and Teychenne, P. F. (1978). Ergot derivatives for Parkinsonism. *Med. J. Aust.* **2**, No. 3 (Spec. Suppl.), 25–26.

Child, D. F., Gordon, H., Mashiter, K. and Joplin, G. F. (1975). Pregnancy, prolactin and pituitary tumours. *Br. med. J.* **4**, 87–89.

Clark, B. J. (1981). Dopamine receptors and the cardiovascular system. *Postgrad. med. J.* **57** (Suppl. 1), 45–54.

Clark, B. J., Scholtysik, G. and Flückiger, E. (1978). Cardiovascular actions of Bromocriptine. *Acta Endocrinol. (Kbh.)* **88** (Suppl. 216), 75–81.

Corenblum, B., Webster, B. R., Mortimer, C. B. and Ezrin, C. (1975). Possible anti-tumor effect of 2-bromo-ergocryptine (CB 154, Sandoz) in two patients with large prolactin secreting pituitary adenomas. *Clin. Res.* **23**, 614A.

Corrodi, H., Fuxe, K., Hökfelt, T., Lindbrink, P. and Ungerstedt, U. (1973). Effect of ergot drugs on central catecholamine neurons: evidence for a stimulation of central dopamine neurons. *J. Pharm. Pharmacol.* **25**, 409–411.

Del Pozo, E. and Lancranjan, I. (1978). Clinical use of drugs modifying the release of anterior pituitory hormones. *In:* "Frontiers in Neuroendocrinology". Vol. 5, (ed. W. F. Ganong and L. Martini), pp. 207–247. New York: Raven Press.

Del Pozo, E. and Maclay, W. P. (1976). Gastrointestinal bleeding in patients on bromocriptine. *Lancet* **II**, 906–907.

Del Pozo, E., Brun Del Re, R., Varga, L. and Friesen, H. (1972). The inhibition of prolactin secretion in man by CB 154 (2 Br-α-ergokryptine). *J. Clin. Endocrinol. Metab.* **35**, 768–771.

Del Pozo, E., Wyss, H., Lancranjan, I., Obolensley, W. and Varga, L. (1976). Prolactin induced luteal insufficiency and its treatment with bromocriptine: preliminary results. *In:* "Ovulation in the Human", (ed. P. G. Crosegari and D. R. Mishell). pp. 297–299. London: Academic Press.

Duvoisin, R. C., Mendoza, M. R., Yahr, M. D. and Sweet, R. D. (1979). Bromocriptine as an adjuvant to levodopa. *In:* "Dopaminergic Ergot Derivatives and Motor Function", (ed. K. Fuxe and D. B. Calne), pp. 329–335. Oxford, New York: Pergamon Press.

Editorial (1971). Human Prolactin. *Br. med. J.* **3**, 201–202.

Flückiger, E. (1972). Drugs and the control of prolactin secretion. "Prolactin and Carcinogenesis". (ed. Boyns, A. R., and Griffiths, K.) pp. 162–171. Cardiff (U.K.): Alpha Omega Alpha Publishing.

Flückiger, E. (1978). Lactation inhibition by ergot drugs. *In:* "Physiology of Mammary Glands", (ed. Yokoyama, A., Mizuno, H., and Nagasawa, H.), pp. 71–82. Tokyo, Japan: Scientific Societies Press.

Flückiger, E., and Vigouret, J. M. (1981). Central dopamine receptors. *Postgrad. med. J.* **57** (Suppl. 1), 55–61.

Flückiger, E., Del Pozo, E., and Von Werder, K. (1982). "Prolactin. Physiology, Pharmacology and Clinical Findings". Monographs on Endocrinology, vol. 23. Berlin, Springer-Verlag.

Franks, S., Jacobs, H. S., Martin, N. and Nabarro, J. D. N. (1978). Hyperprolactinaemia and impotence. *Clin. Endocrinol. (Oxf)* **8**, 277–287.

Frantz, A. G. and Kleinberg, D. L. (1970). Prolactin: Evidence that it is separate from growth hormone in human blood. *Science* **170**, 745–747.

Geschwind, I. I. (1972). Introduction. "Prolactin and Carcinogenesis". (ed. Boyns, A. R., and Griffiths, K.), pp. 1–3. Cardiff (U.K.): Alpha Omega Alpha Publishing.

Griffith, R. W., Turkalj, I. and Braun, P. (1978). Outcome of pregnancy in mothers treated with bromocriptine. *Br. J. Clin. Pharmacol.* **7**, 393–396.

Hafiez, A. A., Bartke, A. and Lloyd, C. W. (1972). The role of testis function: the synergistic effects of prolactin and luteinizing hormone on the incorporation of 1-14-C acetate into testosterone and cholesterol by testes from hypophysectomized rats *in vitro*. *J. Endocrinol.* **53**, 223–230.

Heuson, J. C., Waelbroeck-van Graver, C. and Legros, N. (1970). Growth inhibition of rat mammary carcinoma and endocrine changes produced by 2-Br-α-ergocryptine, a suppressor of lactation and nidation. *Eur. J. Cancer,* **6**, 353–356.

Heuson, J. C., Coune, A. and Staquet (1972). Clinical trial of 2-Br-α-Ergocryptine (CB-154) in advanced breast cancer. *Eur. J. Cancer* **8**, 155–156.

Hökfelt, T. and Fuxe, K. (1972). On the morphology and the neuroendocrine role of the hypothalamic catecholamine neurones. "Brain-Endocrine Interaction. Median Eminence: Structure and Function". (ed. Knigge, K. M., Scott, D. E., and Weindl, A.), pp. 181–223. Basel, Karger.

Hwang, P., Guyda, H. and Friesen, H. (1971). A radioimmunoassay for human prolactin. *Proc. Natl. Acad. Sci. USA* **68**, 1902–1906.

Hwang, P., Guyda, H. and Friesen, H. G. (1972). Purification of human prolactin. *J. Biol. Chem.* **247**, 1955–1958.

Krupp, P. (1981). Pleuropulmonary changes during long-term bromocriptine treatment for Parkinsons Disease. (The manufacturer's reply). *Lancet* **I**, 44.

Landolt, A. M., Wuethrich, R. and Fellmann, H. (1979). Regression of pituitary prolactinoma after treatment with bromocriptine. *Lancet* **I**, 1082–1083.

Lewis, U. J., Singh, R. N. P., Sinha, Y. N. and Vanderlaan, W. P. (1971). Electrophoretic evidence for human prolactin. *J. Clin. Endocrinol.* **33**, 153–156.

Liuzzi, A., Chiodini, P. G., Botalla, L., Cremascoli, G. and Silvestrini, F. (1972). Inhibitory effect of L-DOPA on GH release in acromegalic patients. *J. Clin. Endocrinol. Metab.* **35**, 941–943.

Liuzzi, A., Chiodini, P. G., Botalla, L., Cremascoli, G., Mueller, E. E. and Silvestrini, F. (1974). Decreased plasma growth hormone (GH) levels in acromegalics following CB 154 (2-Br-α-ergokryptine) administration. *J. Clin. Endocrinol. Metab.* **38**, 910–912.

Loew, D. M., Vigouret, J. M. and Jaton, A. L. (1976). Neuropharmacological investigations with two ergot alkaloids, Hydergine and bromocriptine. *Postgrad. med. J.* **52** (Suppl. 1), 40–46.

Lu, K. H., Huang, H. T., Chen, M., Kurcz, M., Mioduszewski, R. and Meites, J. (1977). Positive feedback by oestrogen and progesterone on LH release in old and young rats. *Proc. Soc. Exp. Biol. Med.* **154**, 82–85.

Lutterbeck, P. M., Pryor, S., Varga, L., and Wenner, R. (1971). Treatment of non-puerperal galactorrhoea with an ergot alkaloid. *Br. med. J.* **3**, 228–229.

Macleod, R. M. (1976), Regulation of prolactin secretion. *In:* "Frontiers in Neuroendocrinology", (ed. Martini, L., and Ganong, W. F.), pp. 169–194. New York: Raven Press.

March, C. M. (1979). Bromocriptine in the treatment of hypogonadism and male impotence. *Drugs* **17**, 349–358.

Marko, M. and Flückiger, E. (1974). Inhibition of spontaneous and induced ovulation in rats by non-steroidal agents. *Experientia* **30**, 1174–1176.

Maurer, R. A. (1980). Dopaminergic inhibition of prolactin synthesis and prolactin messenger RNA accumulation in cultured pituitary cells. *J. Biol. Chem.* **255**, 8092–8097.

Maurer, R. A. (1981). Transcriptional regulation of the prolactin gene by ergocryptine and cyclic AMP. *Nature* **294**, 94–97.

Meites, J., Huang, H. H. and Riegle, G. D. (1976). Relation of the hypothalamopituitary-gonadal system to decline of reproductive functions in aging female rats. *In:* "Hypothalamus and Endocrine Functions" (ed. Labrie, F., Meites, J. and Pelletier, G.) New York and London: Plenum Press.

Morgan, L., Barrett, A. and Hobbs, J. R. (1976). Bromocryptine and growth hormone. *Lancet* **I**, 195.

Muller, G. G. and Kirk, R. W. (1969). *In:* "Small Animal Dermatology", pp. 300–302 and 318–320. Philadelphia, London and Toronto: W. B. Saunders.

Pasteels, J. L. (1973). Introduction. "Human Prolactin". (ed. Pasteels, J. L. and Robyn, C.), pp. X–XIII. Amsterdam: Excerpta Medica.

Pasteels, J. L., Danguy, A., Trerotte, M., and Ectors, F. (1971). Inhibition de la sécrétion de prolactine par l'ergocornine et la 2-Br-α-ergokryptine: Action directe sur l'hypophyse en culture. *Ann. Endocrinol. (Paris)*, **32**, 188–192.

Pelkonen, R., Ylikahri, R. and Karonen, S. L. (1980). Bromocriptine treatment of patients with acromegaly resistant to conventional therapy. *Clin. Endocrinol.* **12**, 219–224.

Rennels, E. G. and Callahan, W. P. (1959). The hormonal basis of pubertal maturation of hair in the albino rat. *Anat. Rec.* **135**, 21–27.

Richardson, B. P. (1973). Evidence for a physiological role of prolactin in osmoregulation in the rat. *Br. J. Pharmacol.* **47**, 623P.

Richardson, B. P. and Luginbuehl, H-R. (1976). The role of prolactin in the development of chronic progressive nephropathy in the rat. *Virchow's Arch.* **370**, 13–16.

Rinne, U. K. (1981). Pleuropulmonary changes during long-term bromocriptine treatment for Parkinsons disease. *Lancet* **I**, 44.

Shelesnyak, M. C. (1954). Ergotoxine inhibition of deciduoma formation and its reversal by progesterone. *Am. J. Physiol.* **179**, 301–304.

Schellekens, L. A., Snuiverink, H. and Van Den Berghe, H., (1977). Chromosomal patterns of children born after induction of ovulation with bromocriptine. *Arzneim.-Forsch. (Drug Res.)* **27**, 2151–2153.

Schneider, H. R., Stadler, P. A., Stuetz, P., Troxler, F. and Seres, J. (1977). Synthese und Eigenschaften von Bromocriptine. *Experientia* **33**, 1412–1413.

Scholtysik, G. (1980). Inhibition of cardiac sympathetic neurotransmission in cats by ergot alkaloids. "Presynaptic Receptors", (ed. Langer, S. Z.), pp. 87–92. Oxford: Pergamon Press.

Theohar, C., Fischer-Cornelssen, Akesson, H. O., Ansari, J., Gerlach, J., Harper, P., Oehman, R., Ose, E. and Stegink, A. J., (1981). Bromocriptine as antidepressant: double blind comparative study with imipramine in psychogenic and endogenous depression. *Curr. ther. Res.* **30**, 830–842.

Thomson, M. J., Garland, M. R. and Archards, J. F. (1973). Hormonal effects on thymidine kinase and thymidylate kinase activity of oestrogen dependent tumors in the rat. *Cancer Res.* **33**, 220–225.

Thorner, M. O., Besser, G. M., Jones, A., Dacie, J., and Jones, A. E. (1975a). Bromocriptine treatment of female infertility: report of 13 pregnancies. *Br. med. J.* **4**, 694–697.

Thorner, M. O., Chait, A., Aitken, M., Bender, G., Bloom, S. R., Mortimer, C. H., Sanders, P., Stuart Mason, A. and Besser, G. M. (1975b). Bromocriptine treatment of acromegaly. *Br. med. J.* **1**, 299–303.

Thorner, M. O., Flückiger, E. and Calne, D. B. (1980). Bromocriptine. "A Clinical and Pharmacological Review". New York: Raven Press.

Turkalj, I., Braun, P. and Krupp, P. (1982). Surveillance of bromocriptine in pregnancy. *J.A.M.A.* **247**, 1589–1591.

Varga, L., Lutterbeck, P. M., Pryor, S., Wenner, R. and Erb, H. (1972). Suppression of puerperal lactation with an ergot alkaloid: A double-blind study. *Br. med. J.* **2**, 743–744.

Varga, L., Wenner, R. and Del Pozo, E. (1973). Treatment of galactorrhoea-amenorrhoea syndrome with Br-ergocryptine (CB 154): Restoration of ovulatory function and fertility. *Am. J. Obstet. Gynecol.* **117**, 75–79.

Wass, J. A. H., Thorner, M. O. and Besser, G. M. (1976a). Digital vasospasm with bromocriptine. *Lancet* **I**, 1135.

Wass, J. A. H., Thorner, M. O., Besser, G. M., Morris, D., Stuart-Mason, A., Liuzzi, A. and Chiodini, P. G. (1976b). Gastrointestinal bleeding in patients on bromocriptine. *Lancet* **II**, 851.

Wass, J. A. H., Thorner, M. O., Charlesworth, M., Moult, P. J. A., Dacie, J. E., Jones, A. E. and Besser, G. M. (1979). Reduction of pituitary tumour size in patients with prolactinomas and acromegaly treated with bromocriptine with or without radiotherapy. *Lancet* **II**, 66–69.

Welsch, C. W. and Gribler, C. (1973). Prophylaxis of Spontaneously developing mammary carcinoma in C3H/HeJ female mice by suppression of prolactin. *Cancer Res.* **33**, 2939–2946.

Welsch, C. W. and Nagasawa, H. (1977). Prolactin and murine mammary tumorigenesis: A Review. *Cancer Res.* **37**, 951–963.

Wigley, R. D. (1970). The aetiology of polyarteritis nodosa: A Review. *New Zealand med. J.* **71**, 151–158.

Yanai, R., and Nagasawa, H. (1970). Effects of ergocornine and 2-Br-α-ergocryptine (CB 154) on the formation of mammary hyperplastic alveolar nodules and the pituitary prolactin levels in mice. *Experientia* **26**, 649–650.

Yanai, R., and Nagasawa, H. (1974). Effect of 2-Br-α-ergocryptine on pituitary synthesis and release of prolactin and growth hormone in rats. *Hormone Res.* **5**, 1–5.

Zeilmaker, G. H., and Carlsen, R. A. (1962). Experimental studies on the effect of ergocornine methanesulfonate on the luteotrophic function of the rat pituitary gland. *Acta Endocrinol. (Kbh)* **41**, 321–335.

# 4

# Cimetidine

R. W. BRIMBLECOMBE and G. B. LESLIE

*Smith Kline and French Research Ltd., The Frythe,*
*Welwyn, Hertfordshire, England*

## I. Summary

Cimetidine, $N''$-cyano-n-methyl-$N'$-2-[(5-methylimidazol-4-yl) methylthio] ethyl guanidine, is a specific competitive histamine $H_2$-receptor antagonist which has been shown to inhibit gastric acid secretion in experimental animals and man. It was synthesized during 1972 and toxicological studies on the compound commenced in 1973. It was first marketed in 1976.

Cimetidine was shown in animal studies to have a very weak anti-androgenic activity and increased the incidence of benign Leydig cell tumours in rats after two years of treatment. Very high doses in dogs caused hypotension and tachycardia and two dogs had centrilobular degeneration and renal tubular nephrosis. Apart from this the compound had no significant toxic effects in long term repeated dose studies and had very low acute toxicity. Clinical experience has also demonstrated the lack of significant adverse effects. Those effects which have been seen are largely idiosyncratic and of very low incidence. Studies carried out prior to the marketing of cimetidine did not predict any carcinogenic potential. Studies instituted post-marketing to investigate a hypothetical causal relationship between cimetidine and gastric cancer have not produced evidence to contradict this conclusion, i.e. there is still no hard evidence to link cimetidine to gastric carcinoma.

## II. Introduction

The antihistaminics developed during the 1940's were specific competitive antagonists of the action of histamine in stimulating the contraction of smooth muscle from organs such as the guinea pig ileum, bronchus and uterus. They did not, however, block all the actions of histamine. They only partially blocked the vasodilator effects of large doses of histamine and they were totally unable to inhibit histamine-induced gastric acid secretion. They also failed to prevent histamine-induced inhibition of the evoked contractions of the rat isolated uterus and histamine-induced increase in the rate of contraction of the isolated guinea pig right atrium.

These facts suggested the existence of more than one type of histamine receptor and in 1964 Dr. J. W. Black initiated a research programme in our laboratories to discover a specific antagonist of histamine at those receptors resistant to the conventional antihistaminic drugs. In 1966 Ash and Schild defined the histamine $H_1$-receptor as that which mediates those responses to histamine which could be antagonized by conventional antihistaminics. Since at that time there were no known antagonists for the other actions of histamine, the receptors involved were left unclassified except as non-$H_1$. These non $H_1$-receptors are now defined as $H_2$-receptors and the programme in our laboratories was designed to find a molecule that would compete with histamine at this $H_2$-receptor site. Such a molecule would have to bind to the receptor more strongly than histamine but should not trigger the usual response.

The starting point for the development of such a molecule was the structure of histamine itself (Fig. 1). Histamine was modified chemically and during the first four years of the programme some 200 compounds were synthesized and tested for their ability to antagonize the actions of histamine on the isolated rat uterus and guinea pig atrium and to inhibit histamine-stimulated gastric acid secretion using the lumen-perfused rat stomach preparation of Ghosh and Schild (1958) as modified by Parsons (1969). This approach ultimately led to the synthesis of burimamide, the first histamine $H_2$-receptor antagonist to be described. Burimamide was shown to inhibit histamine-induced gastric acid secretion in man (Wyllie et al., 1972) but the compound was inadequately active orally and a more potent compound was sought.

Stepwise modifications led to the synthesis of metiamide which was some 8 to 9 times more potent than burimamide in vitro and some 4 to 6 times more potent in vivo. Metiamide was shown to be highly effective in reducing gastric acid secretion and proved to be of therapeutic value in the treatment of duodenal ulcer (Celestin et al., 1975). In a small number of patients receiving metiamide a reversible granulocytopenia was observed (Forrest et al., 1975). It was considered that this effect could be related to the presence of the thiourea group in metiamide and clinical research therefore continued with one of the non-thiourea antagonists already in development. The replacement of the thiourea by cyanoguanidine in 1972 produced cimetidine which was more potent than metiamide and was the first histamine $H_2$-receptor antagonist to be marketed (1976).

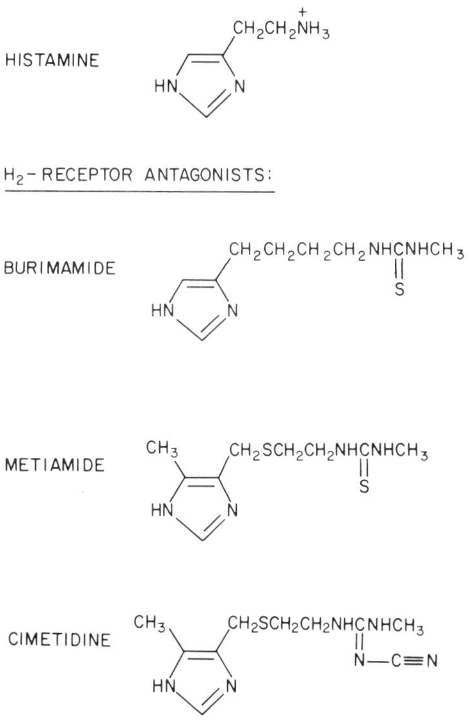

HISTAMINE

$CH_2CH_2\overset{+}{N}H_3$

HN N

$H_2$– RECEPTOR ANTAGONISTS:

BURIMAMIDE

$CH_2CH_2CH_2CH_2NHCNHCH_3$
$\overset{\parallel}{S}$

HN N

METIAMIDE

$CH_3$   $CH_2SCH_2CH_2NHCNHCH_3$
$\overset{\parallel}{S}$

HN N

CIMETIDINE

$CH_3$   $CH_2SCH_2CH_2NHCNHCH_3$
$\overset{\parallel}{N-C\equiv N}$

HN N

FIG. 1. The chemical structures of histamine and three histamine $H_2$-receptor antagonists.

## III. Preclinical data

### A. Pharmacology

The pharmacological properties of cimetidine have been described by Brimblecombe and Duncan (1977) and by Brimblecombe *et al.*, (1978). Apart from its properties demonstrably due to antagonism of histamine at the $H_2$-receptor, cimetidine has little effect on other physiological systems. At doses some 10 to 20 times those required to inhibit acid secretion, cimetidine inhibited spontaneous gastric motility in the rat. Very high doses of cimetidine can cause vasodilatation and hypotension (Brimblecombe and Duncan, 1977). The mechanisms of these actions are not understood.

### B. Acute Toxicology

The acute toxicity of cimetidine following oral, intravenous, and intra-

TABLE 1. Acute $LD_{50}$ values for cimetidine

| Species | Route | $LD_{50}$ |
|---------|-------|-----------|
| Mouse | iv | 150 |
| Mouse | ip | 470 |
| Mouse | po | 2600 |
| Rat | iv | 106 |
| Rat | ip | 650 |
| Rat | po | 5000 |
| Hamster | ip | 880 |
| Hamster | po | 4000 |

Groups of 10 animals, of each sex, were dosed with cimetidine in solution. The $LD_{50}$ values were calculated for each sex group using the method of Litchfield and Wilcoxon (1949); the results quoted are the average of these values. iv, intravenous; ip, intraperitoneal; po, per os.

peritoneal dosing of a solution has been studied in mice, rats and hamsters (Table 1). In dogs the $LD_{50}$ value after oral dosing of solution was approximately 2.6 g/kg.

## C. Sub-Acute and Chronic Toxicology

Repeated dose oral toxicity studies began in our laboratories in 1973 using rats and dogs dosed seven days per week. The early toxicity studies have been described by Leslie and Walker (1977). In rats repeated dose studies of up to 24 months duration with daily doses up to 950 mg/kg/day (680 times the acute intraduodenal $ID_{50}$ for inhibition of stimulated gastric acid secretion in the anaesthetized rat) showed very few adverse effects. Excess salivation was observed after dosing in the top dose group and perineal soiling was also commonly seen. These effects were attributed to the unpleasant taste of the dosing solution and the urine. No significant differences between the groups were observed in body weight, food consumption, blood chemistry, urinalysis, or ophthalmoscopy. Slightly low haemoglobin concentrations were observed in the female rats during the 30-day study but not in subsequent studies; no other haematological abnormalities were seen. In three-, six-, 12- and 24-month studies, the livers of the top dose group animals were heavier than those of the controls. After 24-months dosing there was a reduction in size and atrophy of the prostates and seminal vesicles of all of the dosed groups. Examination of other tissues revealed no histopathological abnormalities attributable to drug treatment. No evidence was seen of any adverse effects on the alimentary canal. Exposure to cimetidine for 24 months did not increase the risk of any malignant neoplasm.

A statistically significant decrease in the incidence of tumours of the pituitary and of the mammary gland and an increased incidence in tumours of the Leydig cells were found when the combined treated groups were compared with the combined control groups (one control group received distilled water and the other group was undosed). The following observations were made: (1) there were no dose–response relationships, and (2) the incidence of these three tumours in the combined treated groups was not significantly different from that in the undosed control group. Additionally, with the tumours of the Leydig cells there was no evidence of an earlier occurrence of tumours in the treated groups. All the Leydig cell tumours were benign.

Table 4.2 summarizes the findings in our oral repeated dose studies in rats. The two year study in rats has been described in detail by Leslie *et al.* (1981).

A second two year study in rats commenced in 1978 using male rats only. The findings confirmed those of our original study. In particular, the slightly increased incidence of Leydig cell tumours and hyperplasia in the treated groups and the reduction in prostate and seminal vesicle weights were again observed. In this second study the histology of the stomach was given particular attention. The lack of any treatment-related changes was confirmed.

In dogs, repeated dose studies of up to 12 months duration have been completed with oral doses up to 504 mg/kg/day (203 times the estimated $ID_{50}$ for inhibition of maximally stimulated gastric acid secretion in the dog). This dose caused marked tachycardia after dosing and a rapid weight loss during the first 2 weeks of the test. The dose was therefore reduced to 336 mg/kg/day from week 9 and was increased in steps until week 12 when the dose was again 504 mg/kg/day. Two dogs receiving this dose had to be killed before the end of the test because of their deteriorating clinical condition. In these two dogs histological examination showed centrilobular degeneration in the liver and renal tubular nephrosis. Both dogs had high serum transaminases and one dog had a high serum alkaline phosphatase in blood samples taken immediately before they were killed. Occasional, but not progressive, elevations of serum transaminases and serum alkaline phosphatase were seen in other dogs in this dose group and minor degenerative changes were observed in the centrilobular areas of the liver in animals killed after the six-month dosing with 504 mg/kg/day. Such changes were not observed at lower doses and, in the top dose group dogs killed after 12 months, no treatment-related histological changes were seen in the liver, despite the biochemical changes observed earlier, indicating that the slight changes seen at six months were not progressive.

Of the dogs killed after the six-month dosing, all of the males receiving cimetidine at all dose levels showed a reduction in the development of the

TABLE 2. Cimetidine: Oral repeated dose studies in rats

| Dose mg/kg | 30-day | 90-day | 6-month | 12-month | 24-month |
|---|---|---|---|---|---|
| 950 | Excessive salivation; slight increase in liver weights; slightly low hemoglobin in females. | Excessive salivation; perineal soiling; slight increase in liver weights. | Excessive salivation; perineal soiling; increase in liver weights; prostates and seminal vesicles lighter than controls. | Excessive salivation perineal soiling; increase in liver weights; prostates and seminal vesicles lighter than controls. | Excess salivation; perineal soiling; increase in liver weights; prostates and seminal vesicles lighter than controls. |
| 378 | Slightly low hemoglobin in females | NAD | Increased liver weight in males; seminal vesicles lighter than controls. | Prostates lighter than controls. | Increased liver weights in males; prostates and seminal vesicles lighter than controls. |
| 150 | NAD | NAD | Increased liver weight in males. | Prostates slightly lighter than controls. | Prostates and seminal vesicles lighter than controls. |

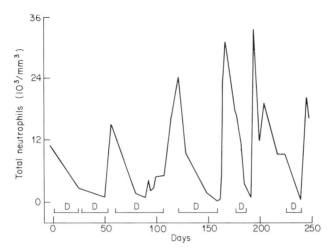

FIG. 2. The effect of dosing with 162 mg/kg metiamide (D) on total neutrophilic count in a susceptible beagle dog.

prostate. In the dogs killed after 1 year the reduction in the size of the prostate was found to have been progressive, although some reduced development of glandular elements was seen in all males in the two higher dose groups and in two of six males receiving 114 mg/kg/day.

Apart from this, the dogs receiving 114 mg/kg/day showed no other effects attributable to cimetidine, and no effects attributable to cimetidine were observed after the 12-month dosing with 41 mg/kg/day. The haematology, differential bone marrow counts, blood chemistry, urinalysis, ophthalmoscopy, electrocardiography and histopathology, including that of the gut, were normal.

In a three-month oral study of metiamide in dogs 2/12 animals dosed at 81 mg/kg/day or more showed reversible granulocytopenia. In the 12-month study in dogs with the same doses of this compound the reversible granulocytopenia was seen in 3/16 animals. An example of the effect is illustrated in Fig. 2. As can be seen, the granulocytopenia is very readily reversed by cessation of dosing. No such effect was seen with cimetidine in any of our dog studies. Cross (1977) has shown that metiamide accumulates in the bone marrow of rats and dogs but cimetidine does not. The thiourea group on metiamide is believed to influence its distribution to the bone marrow. Table 3 summarizes the findings in our oral repeated dose dog studies.

In 1976 we commenced a study administering cimetidine orally to eight male and four female dogs at a dose level of 144 mg/kg/day. After seven

TABLE 3. Cimetidine: oral repeated dose studies in dogs

| Dose mg/kg | 3-month | 6-month | 12-month |
|---|---|---|---|
| 504 | | Transient tachycardia and rapid weight loss (early weeks); slight liver damage; small prostates (30% of controls). One killed (liver and kidney damage). | Transient tachycardia and rapid weight loss (early weeks); no liver damage; small prostates (20% of controls). One killed (liver and kidney damage). |
| 333 | Transient tachycardia and slight weight loss (early weeks); small prostates (40% of controls). | Transient tachycardia (early weeks); small prostates (38% of controls). | Transient tachycardia (early weeks); small prostates (36% of controls). |
| 144 | | Small prostates (42% of controls). | Small prostates (48% of controls). |
| 112 | Slightly small prostates (60% of controls). | | |
| 41 | | Slightly small prostates (64% of controls). | NAD |
| 37 | NAD | | |

years of dosing we have seen no evidence of treatment-related effects on haematology, clinical biochemistry, urinalysis, electrocardiography or clinical condition. Biopsies of gastric mucosa taken during endoscopy in months 41, 47, 53, 59, 65, 71, 77 and 84 have shown no changes attributable to cimetidine treatment (Crean *et al.*, 1981a, b; Whitehead and Leslie, 1983).

## D. Reproductive Toxicology

Teratological studies have been completed in the rat, rabbit and mouse at oral doses up to 950 mg/kg/day. No significant adverse effects were seen.

Fertility tests in male and female rats have also been completed with oral doses of up to 950 mg/kg/day. Mating performance and fertility were not impaired. All offspring of dosed males were normal and there were no dose-related effects on litter parameters. In dosed females there was no effect on oestrous cycles, mating performance, fertility, maternal weight gain or perinatal behaviour and no effects on pre- or post-implantation losses, litter size, viability, or foetal development. In all naturally delivered litters there was no dose-related effect on survival, and weight gain in the young was not affected.

In peri- and postnatal studies, rats were dosed at up to 950 mg/kg/day. There was no effect on maternal weight gain, perinatal behaviour in the parents, litter size and weight, or on physical and behavioural development in the offspring. No reduction in locomotor activity was seen in the offspring. No effect was seen on mating performance, fertility, or litter parameters when the $F_1$ generation reproduced.

## E. Anti-androgenicity

Since cimetidine was shown to have a weak anti-androgenic activity in repeated dose studies in rats and dogs it has been subject to further investigations to quantify this action. It has been shown to have no detectable oestrogenic activity in the immature rat using the assay method described by Hisaw (1959) but has been shown to have weak anti-androgenic activity in immature rats dosed daily with testosterone. Cimetidine has also been shown to antagonize the effects of exogenous testosterone on the prostates and seminal vesicles of young castrate rats. It is well known that the differentiation of the genital organs in male foetuses is influenced by the endogenous testosterone already produced during embryonic development (Wiesner, 1934; Jost, 1947). Active anti-androgens block the testosterone effect in the critical phase of differentiation (Neumann *et al.*, 1965) in both the rat and the rabbit but the phalluses of the male foetuses in all our reproductive studies showed no evidence of feminization.

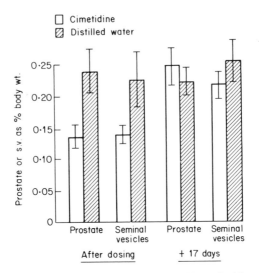

FIG. 3. The effect of cimetidine given orally at 900 mg/kg/day for 35 days, on prostate and seminal vesicle (s.v.) weights in rats.

The effect of cimetidine in retarding the development of the prostate and seminal vesicles in rats is reversible. Rats aged eight months dosed orally for 35 days with either cimetidine at a dose of 950 mg/kg/day or distilled water were divided into two groups: one group was killed at the end of the dosing period and the other 17 days later without further dosing. The sizes of the prostates and seminal vesicles are shown in Fig. 3. Similar results were obtained in rats aged two months at the start of the experiment. The differences between the prostate weights and seminal vesicle weights of the cimetidine-treated animals and distilled water controls were statistically significant immediately after the end of dosing but were not statistically significant after the 17-day period without further dosing in rats of either age group.

Sivelle *et al.*, (1982) showed that the anti-androgenic action of cimetidine is very weak. When calculated on a molar basis the dose of cimetidine needed to inhibit the action of testosterone propionate on the ventral prostate and seminal vesicles of castrate rats was some 543 times that of cyproterone acetate and 16 times that of spironolactone. These workers also demonstrated that other, more potent, histamine $H_2$-receptor antagonists were not anti-androgenic. It is clear, therefore, that the anti-androgenic activity of cimetidine does not involve histamine $H_2$ receptors. Sivelle *et al.* also showed that cimetidine inhibited the androgenic activity of 5α-dihydro-testosterone (DHT). Thus its anti-androgenic activity is not a consequence of preventing the conversion of testosterone to its more active metabolite. Cimetidine also prevented the binding of $^3$H-DHT to the androgen receptor of the rat ventral prostate and they concluded that the anti-androgenic activity was a consequence of this interaction.

## F. Drug Interactions

A number of acute interaction studies have been carried out with cimetidine and a wide range of therapeutic substances. The effects of a fixed dose of some test agents on the acute $LD_{50}$ of cimetidine in rats and mice are listed in Table 4. None of the agents increased the acute toxicity of cimetidine. The test agents used in this study were chlorpheniramine, propantheline, mepyramine, atropine, hydroxyzine, ampicillin, cephalothin, warfarin and heparin. In a second series of studies the effects of simultaneous administration in the rat of combinations of cimetidine and test agents in fixed clinical ratios were studied. No significant interactions with cimetidine were seen (Table 5) using oral administration of atropine, trifluoperazine, chlordiazepoxide, propantheline, isopropamide, phenobarbitone, diazepam, or meprobamate. When administered intravenously, three test agents in combination with cimetidine showed a small significant enhancement of acute toxicity. These were pethidine, thiopentone and propranolol. Other test agents—suxamethonium, tubocurarine, noradrenaline, lignocaine, hydralazine, methyldopa and adrenaline—showed no evidence of acute interactions.

## G. Mutagenicity/Nitrosation

In the Ames test for bacterial mutagenicity, cimetidine is negative at up to 5000 $\mu$g per plate in *Salmonella typhimurium* strains TA 1535, TA 1538, TA 98 and TA 100. However, recent controversy over a possible hypothetical association between cimetidine administration and the development of gastric carcinoma led to an interest in the possible nitrosation of cimetidine and to studies of the properties of its nitrosated derivative.

It has been shown that *in vitro* cimetidine reacts with excess nitrite under strongly acidic conditions (2M HC1) to form a mono-N-nitroso derivative known as N-nitrosocimetidine (Foster *et al.*, 1980; Bavin *et al.*, 1980). The rate of this reaction is pH dependent, with the initial rate dropping by a factor of about ten for each pH unit rise. N-Nitrosocimetidine is positive in the Ames test strains TA 100 and TA 1535 at 100 to 555 $\mu$g per plate (Brimblecombe, 1980). Similarly Pool *et al.*, (1979) reported that N-nitrosocimetidine induces DNA damage in repair-deficient *E. coli* strains at 100 $\mu$g per plate. Cimetidine itself showed no activity.

TABLE 4. Drug interaction studies: effect of a fixed dose of test agent on $LD_{50}$ of cimetidine

| Species | Cimetidine Route | Test Agent | Route and Timing[c] | Test agent Dose mg/kg | $LD_{50}$ Cimetidine Alone mg/kg | $LD_{50}$ in Combination mg/kg | Relative Toxicity (95% Confidence Limits) |
|---|---|---|---|---|---|---|---|
| Mouse | Oral | Chlorpheniramine Maleate | Oral P | 50 | 1970 | 1220 | 1.61[b] |
| | Oral | Chlorpheniramine Maleate | Oral P | 5 | 2320 | 1670 | 1.39[b] |
| | Oral | Propantheline Bromide | Oral P | 200 | 2380 | 1540 | 1.55[b] |
| | Oral | Mepyramine Maleate | Oral P | 90 | 2380 | 1600 | 1.59[b] |
| | I.V. | Chlorpheniramine Maleate | I.V. S | 1 | 106 | 102 | 1.40[a] |
| Rat | Oral | Chlorpheniramine Maleate | Oral P | 50 | 4770 | 3200 | Not parallel lines but significantly decreased $LD_{50}$[b] |
| | Oral | Atropine Sulphate | Oral S | 37.8 | 3566 | 2615 | 1.36 (1.03–1.97)[b] |
| | I.V. | Digoxin | Oral S | 2.4 | 87.9 | 96.4 | 0.91 (0.77–1.08)[a] |
| | I.V. | Hydrocortisone Sodium Succinate | I.V. S | 86 | 104.9 | 111.9 | 0.94 (0.81–1.07)[a] |
| | I.V. | Furosemide | I.V. S | 24 | 101.7 | 101.9 | 1.00 (0.81–1.22)[a] |
| | I.V. | Hydroxyzine Hydrochloride | I.M. S | 100 | 122.2 | 137.7 | 0.89 (0.76–1.05)[a] |
| | I.V. | Sodium Ampicillin | I.V. S | 1279.3 | 113.2 | 122.3 | 0.93 (0.83–1.08)[a] |
| | I.V. | Sodium Cephalothin | I.V. S | 635 | 105.2 | 93.4 | 1.13 (0.98–1.34)[a] |
| | I.V. | Sodium Warfarin | I.V. S | 12 | 107.7 | 99.0 | 1.09 (0.92–1.33)[a] |
| | I.V. | Sodium Heparin | I.V. S | 300 | 119.9 | 118.1 | 1.02 (0.84–1.26)[a] |

[a] $LD_{50}$ of cimetidine in combination with test agent not significantly different from $LD_{50}$ of cimetidine alone.  [b] $LD_{50}$ of cimetidine in combination with test agent significantly less than $LD_{50}$ of cimetidine alone.
[c] P = Test drug administered 30 mins before cimetidine; S = Test drug administered simultaneously with cimetidine.

TABLE 5. Drug interaction studies: effect of simultaneous administration of combination of cimetidine and test agent in the rat in fixed clinical ratio

| Test Agent | Dose Ratio Cimetidine:[c] Test Agent | $LD_{50}$ mg/kg | Relative Toxicity[a] (95% Confidence Limits) |
|---|---|---|---|
| *Route: ORAL* | | | |
| Atropine Sulphate | Cimetidine alone | 2492.6 | |
| | 12:1 | 1793.3 | 0.85 (0.61–1.20)[b] |
| | 24:1 | 2081.1 | 0.93 (0.68–1.27)[b] |
| | 48:1 | 1908.1 | 0.80 (0.58–1.10)[b] |
| | 143:1 | 2815.0 | 1.13 (0.83–1.55)[b] |
| | Test Agent alone | 725.6 | |
| Chlordiazepoxide Hydrochloride | Cimetidine alone | 4202.0 | |
| | 25:1 | 3611.9 | 1.04 (0.80–1.37)[b] |
| | Test Agent alone | 640.0 | |
| Diazepam | Cimetidine alone | 2606.0 | |
| | 25:1 | 2689.0 | 1.05 (0.74–1.50)[b] |
| | Test Agent alone | 1713.0 | |
| Isopropamide Iodide | Cimetidine alone | 4641.0 | |
| | 50:1 | 3499.0 | 1.30 (0.97–1.95)[b] |
| | Test Agent alone | 2354.0 | |
| Meprobamate | Cimetidine alone | 2952.0 | |
| | 1:2 | 1094.0 | 0.82 (0.60–1.11)[b] |
| | Test Agent alone | 1055.0 | |
| Phenobarbitone Sodium | Cimetidine alone | 2823.4 | |
| | 8.3:1 | 1401.6 | 1.17 (0.84–1.62)[b] |
| | Test Agent alone | 208.3 | |

*continued overleaf*

TABLE 5. *Continued*

| Test Agent | Dose Ratio Cimetidine:[c] Test Agent | LD$_{50}$ mg/kg | Relative Toxicity[a] (95% Confidence Limits) |
|---|---|---|---|
| Propantheline Bromide | Cimetidine alone 14:1 | 3315.0 2496.0 | 0.97 (0.74–1.28)[b] |
| | Test Agent alone | 621.5 | |
| Trifluoperazine Dihydrochloride | Cimetidine alone 250:1 | 3253.0 2439.0 | 1.32 (0.98–1.78)[b] |
| | Test Agent alone | 909.0 | |
| *Route i.v.* | | | |
| Adrenaline | Cimetidine alone 266.7:1 | 106.7 111.3 | 0.96 (0.85–1.08)[b] |
| | Test Agent alone | 3.8 | |
| Hydralazine Hydrochloride | Cimetidine alone 10:1 | 111.0 99.4 | 1.04 (0.87–1.23)[b] |
| | Test Agent alone | 40.2 | |
| Lignocaine hydrochloride | Cimetidine alone 1:0.75 | 113.3 34.9 | 1.10 (0.85–1.43)[b] |
| | Test Agent alone | 16.2 | |
| Methyldopa hydrochloride | Cimetidine alone 1:5 | 114.6 170.9 | 1.10 (0.96–1.27)[b] |
| | Test Agent alone | 166.5 | |
| Noradrenaline bitartrate | Cimetidine alone 5.9:1 | 103.6 0.42 | 1.45 (0.85–2.49)[c] |
| | Test Agent alone | 0.09 | |

| Test agent | Treatment | LD₅₀ | | Relative toxicity (95% confidence limits) |
|---|---|---|---|---|

| Test agent | Treatment | Value | Relative toxicity |
|---|---|---|---|
| Pethidine hydrochloride | Cimetidine alone | 122.4 | |
| | 2.7:1 | 163.4 | $1.39\,(1.16–1.66)^{d}$ |
| | Test Agent alone | 106.4 | |
| Propranolol hydrochloride | Cimetidine alone | 101.9 | |
| | 133.3:1 | 114.9 | $1.16\,(1.01–1.33)^{d}$ |
| | Test Agent alone | 30.9 | |
| Sodium Thiopentone | Cimetidine alone | 112.1 | |
| | 1:2.5 | 57.5 | $1.24\,(1.04–1.47)^{d}$ |
| | Test Agent alone | 37.5 | |
| Suxamethonium chloride | Cimetidine alone | 129.3 | |
| | 5.3:1 | 3.42 | $1.14\,(0.97–1.34)^{b}$ |
| | Test Agent only | 0.49 | |
| Tubocurarine chloride | Cimetidine alone | 119.4 | |
| | 44:1 | 3.51 | $0.98\,(0.79–1.23)^{b}$ |
| | Test Agent alone | 0.08 | |

[a] Relative toxicity calculated by Finney's Analysis of Mixture method (1971). [b] No significant interaction between cimetidine and test agent. [c] Cimetidine was administered as the hydrochloride salt in all studies in which the drug was administered i. v. The ratio was calculated on the dose expressed as the base. [d] LD₅₀ of cimetidine in combination with test agent significantly higher than predicted. [e] Lines not parallel but no significant interaction on 50% region of the lines.

Attention has been drawn to the apparent structural similarity between N-nitrosocimetidine and N-methyl-N'-nitro-N-nitrosoguanidine (MNNG). The latter compound is a gastric carcinogen in some species of experimental animal (Sugimura and Fujimura, 1967). This has led to a number of studies comparing the properties of the two compounds.

In the Ames test using *S. typhimurium* and in the *E. coli* test referred to above, MNNG was considerably more active than N-nitrosocimetidine. Jensen and Magee (1981) studied the *in vitro* reaction of MNNG and N-nitro socimetidine with DNA and concluded that they were equipotent as methylating agents. Various other workers have confirmed in different test situations that N-nitrosocimetidine reacts with or damages DNA. Where comparisons have been made, N-nitrosocimetidine was never more active and was usually considerably less active than MNNG.

In an *in vivo* study Gombar *et al.* (1981) administered [14]C-labelled cimetidine, N-nitro socimetidine or MNNG orally to rats. The animals were killed twelve hours later and DNA was isolated from various tissues. No methylation of DNA was detected in cimetidine-treated rats. Methylation of DNA from most tissues was observed following MNNG or N-nitro-socimetidine administration but in all cases MNNG produced a higher level of alkylation than did N-nitro socimetidine (3 to 50 times depending on the tissue).

While all these studies are of interest, their relevance to the production of human gastric carcinoma remains a matter for controversy and debate. Somewhat more relevant are long-term feeding studies in which N-nitro-socimetidine has been given in large doses to animals. Evidence to date indicates a lack of carcinogenicity. Eisenbrand (1981) reported that there was no evidence of carcinogenesis in rats given 500 mg/kg N-nitro-socimetidine twice a week for one year (i.e. a *total* dose of about 5–10 g per rat). In contrast Schoental (1966) reported that tumours were found within a year in rats treated with a *total* dose of 10–50 mg per rat of MNNG comprising 3 to 5 doses spread over several months.

It is also convenient at this point to discuss studies in man which are relevant to the issue of a possible association between cimetidine administration and gastric carcinoma. Apart from the possibility that cimetidine could be nitrosated, there is a second hypothesis which proposes that in the hypochlorhydric stomach bacterial colonization can occur. If the bacteria include nitrate-reducing organisms than elevated nitrite levels could lead to a faster nitrosation of amines from food-stuffs and hence to increased levels of total N-nitroso compounds, some of which could be carcinogenic.

There are now many studies which show that when the pH of the gastric juice is around 4 or higher then viable bacteria can be isolated and these usually include nitrate-reducing organisms. There are also a number of studies, well exemplified by that of Reed *et al.* (1981), in which samples of gastric juice have been taken following cimetidine administration and where concentrations of nitrite and nitrosamines and bacterial counts have been elevated. A correlation is claimed between gastric pH and nitrite and nitrosamine concentrations. However, in this and other similar studies only single fasting gastric aspirates were obtained and the patients had received cimetidine (200 mg orally) one to four hours before the aspirates were taken. Hence, the pH was inevitably high and bacteria were inevitably present. The method used to determine "nitrosamine" concentrations is unlikely to detect nitrosamides which are considered to be direct acting carcinogens.

Other studies have been designed to monitor intragastric conditions over the full 24 h period in subjects on full dose (3 × 200 and 1 × 400 mg) and maintenance dose (400 mg nocte) cimetidine. In a recent study by Milton-Thompson *et al.* (1982) eight volunteer subjects were studied before and after two weeks of treatment with 1 g per day cimetidine and after a further two weeks of treatment with 400 mg at night. Gastric juice samples were taken at either half-hourly or hourly intervals. Although nitrite and bacterial levels tended to rise with pH, high ph values occurred only transiently even in the cimetidine-treated subjects. Thus there was not a permanent colonization of the stomach by bacteria. N-Nitroso compounds were analysed by a new method (Bavin *et al.*, 1981) which measures total compounds, not just the stable ones. Concentrations of these compounds fluctuated considerably but they were not affected by cimetidine treatment and contrary to the findings by Reed *et al.* (1981) they did not correlate with pH, nitrite or bacterial counts.

## H. Pharmacokinetics and Metabolism

In rats and dogs cimetidine is rapidly absorbed and is mainly excreted unchanged in the urine, the plasma half-life being about one hour. The principal metabolite in both species is formed by oxidation of the side chain sulphur to give the sulphoxide, which is less active than the parent compound as an $H_2$-receptor antagonist (Taylor *et al.*, 1978).

The kinetics, absorption, distribution, metabolism and elimination of cimetidine in man and experimental animals have been discussed by Griffiths *et al.* (1977). In man the compound is absorbed efficiently from the gut after oral administration. A large proportion of an orally administered dose was found unchanged in the urine with the remainder being represented by more polar metabolites. The bioavailability of a dose given by mouth was about 70% of the availability of an intravenous bolus injection. When given intravenously, doses of cimetidine were also excreted largely as unchanged drug. Data from blood concentration measurements indicated that the disposition of cimetidine was initially more rapid into a second kinetic compartment. After equilibration, clearance of cimetidine was mainly by the kidney; the half-life of elimination was just under two hours.

These data obtained for man are in good agreement with the corresponding results from rat and dog, the species used in the toxicological studies. In all three species cimetidine is well absorbed after oral dosing, producing concentrations of unchanged drug in blood and urine greater than the concentration of any metabolite.

In all three species the sulphoxide represented the major metabolite; no minor metabolites were found in human urine that had not been identified previously in the urine of rats and dogs although the relative proportions were slightly different. In all three species, following intravenous administration of radiolabelled compound, a small amount of material derived from cimetidine was excreted in the faeces indicating that routes of excretion other than the kidney are available. These results indicate that the use of rats and dogs as animal models for man in long-term toxicity tests is justified on kinetic and metabolic grounds.

The distribution of cimetidine has been studied in rats. It is widely distributed through virtually all tissues except the central nervous system. Cross (1977) has shown that it is rapidly eliminated from all tissues, although in whole body autoradiography studies very small amounts of radioactivity are detectable in liver, kidney and adrenal cortex for about seven days after dosing.

# IV. Clinical experience

Cimetidine was marketed in the *UK* in November 1976 under the name "Tagamet". "Tagamet" is currently approved for marketing in 122 countries and has been given to well over 20,000,000 patients.

Between November 1976 and September 1980 the Committee on the Safety of Medicines had received 2370 reports on adverse events associated with cimetidine. During this period about a million patients in the UK had been treated with cimetidine. The incidence of adverse events associated with cimetidine treatment, therefore, is very low as would have been predicted from the toxicological studies.

## A. Acute Toxicity

This has not been a problem. Acute overdosage of up to 100 tablets (20 g) has been reported several times with no significant ill effects (Illingworth and Jarvie, 1979).

## B. Mental Confusion

Reversible confusional states have occurred, usually in elderly or already very ill patients (e.g., those with renal failure). The cause of this is presumed to be a consequence of the increased permeability of the blood–brain barrier to cimetidine in these patients. Flind *et al.* (1980) reviewed the Smith, Kline and French (SKF) worldwide data available in mid 1978 on the incidence of confusion and other reports of CNS disturbances. There were 57 such reports and of 44 providing enough information only 9 were under age 65, or were without serious concomitant illness or other therapy to account for their abnormal mental state. In these cases the impaired mental state tended to improve when cimetidine was withdrawn.

## C. Endocrinological Effects

Gynaecomastia was reported in clinical trials of cimetidine prior to marketing (Sharpe and Hawkins, 1977). Flind and Rowley-Jones (1982) reported that the incidence of gynaecomastia is between 0.1 and 0.2% of patients treated. Clinically the gynaecomastia is usually reversible and in the majority of cases appears to be of nuisance value only. It is not associated with any abnormalities in plasma hormone levels. In particular, although prolactin levels are consistently transiently raised after intravenous bolus injection of cimetidine (200 mg or more) they are unaffected by normal oral dosing (Burland *et al.*, 1979). It appears probable that gynaecomastia follows an idiosyncratic local alteration in oestrogen/androgen balance at the end organ. The weak anti-androgenic effect of cimetidine has led to speculation about the possibility of male impotence or infertility although there was no suggestion of such effects in rats treated with very high doses. Flind and Rowley-Jones (1982) summarizing the reports of impotence received by SKF (UK) up to May 1981 concluded that there was no evidence that cimetidine is associated with a higher incidence of impotence than could be expected in the general population.

Van Thiel *et al.* (1979) reported that in seven male patients cimetidine treatment was associated with a 30% reduction in sperm count. This work has been criticized on a number of grounds by Flind and Rowley-Jones (1982) and a carefully organized, double-blind, placebo controlled study in 30 normal volunteers by Enzman *et al.* (1981) has shown that cimetidine does not inhibit sperm production nor decrease the biological activity of sperm. Enzman *et al.* also found that cimetidine had no effect on serum concentrations of FSH, LH, prolactin, testosterone or dihydrotestosterone.

## D. Acute Pancreatitis

This is a very rare idiosyncratic adverse effect. To March 1981 SKF (UK) had received seven reports of patients in whom acute pancreatitis had occurred on treatment with cimetidine. In such cases the pancreatitis resolved rapidly with conventional treatment when cimetidine was discontinued (Rowley-Jones and Flind, 1981).

## E. Interstitial Nephritis

There has been a very rare incidence of interstitial nephritis, reversed on withdrawal of cimetidine. Five reports of this complication were received during 1978 in the U.S.A. (Flind *et al.*, 1980). The overall incidence of this reversible effect is less than one in a million patients.

## F. White Blood Cell Disorders

Since metiamide was found to cause granulocytopenia and because of the suggestion that there are $H_2$-receptors on bone marrow stem cells (Byron, 1977), particular attention has been paid to examining reports of blood dyscrasias. Davis *et al.* (1980) reported a worldwide total of over 100 cases of white cell disorders. In only one of these, however, was no other factor found which could have contributed to the changes which occurred. By February 1981 there were 192 worldwide reports of a fall in white cell counts associated with the drug (Rowley-Jones and Flind, 1981) by which time it was estimated that over 11 million patients had received cimetidine and in only two cases were there no other factors such as other drugs or serious concomitant illness present. It is considered likely, therefore, that cimetidine *per se* has no effect on bone marrow although there is a possibility that administration to a patient with an already compromised bone marrow could lead to an adverse effect. Even in these circumstances, however, the complication is unlikely.

## G. Drug Interactions

Cimetidine can interfere with the elimination of drugs in which oxidation is a significant part of the metabolic pathway (Rowley-Jones and Flind, 1981). Interactions with only two types of drugs whose elimination is affected in this way is considered to be potentially serious. The effects of warfarin and acenocoumarol are potentiated (Serlin *et al.*, 1979) and close monitoring of patients on cimetidine receiving oral anti-coagulants is recommended. Neuvonen *et al.* (1980) showed that cimetidine could increase mean serum phenytoin concentrations by as much as 63% and for a drug with such a narrow therapeutic index this could be of clinical consequence.

A number of other drugs have their elimination significantly affected, e.g. diazepam, chlordiazepoxide, propranolol, chlormethiazole and caffeine, but none of these is likely to cause problems clinically.

# H. Post Marketing Surveillance

Soon after the beginning of marketing of cimetidine large scale postmarketing surveillance studies began in the U.K. and the U.S.A. Colin-Jones *et al.* (1981) have described the U.K. study which was designed to investigate 2500 recipients of cimetidine at each of four centres with the same number of matched controls. The results of this study are not yet available.

The preliminary results of the U.S.A. postmarketing surveillance programme have been described by Gifford *et al.* (1980). This study was begun seven months after cimetidine was approved for marketing in the U.S.A. Adverse effects data on 9907 patients were collected in the first phase. 557 adverse effects were reported in 442 patients (4.4%). The incidences of adverse effects are listed in Table 6. Gastro-intestinal effects were the most common. No adverse effects were found which had not previously been reported in investigational studies or by the spontaneous adverse-reaction reporting system. Table 7 summarizes the total number of adverse effects reported in a follow up phase carried out six months after the initial phase. It is based on data obtained from 7911 questionnaires. Adverse effects reported during the first phase are not included. During the study, over 50% of the patients were on therapy for more than three months.

# V. Conclusions

Toxicity tests, and other tests relevant to safety, are carried out with a potential new drug prior to its clinical evaluation to ensure, with as much certainty as possible, that administration to man is likely to present minimal hazard. Additionally, the toxicity tests should identify target organs and tissues for possible adverse effects of the drug. Particular attention can then be paid to monitoring these organs and tissues in the human studies.

TABLE 6. Most frequently reported adverse effects in 9,907 patients receiving therapy with "Tagamet"

| Adverse effects | Percentages of patients | Adverse effects | Percentages of patients |
|---|---|---|---|
| Diarrhoea | 1.0 | Gynaecomastia | 0.2 |
| Nausea and vomiting | 0.8 | Constipation | 0.2 |
| Rash, hives pruritis | 0.4 | Gas | 0.2 |
| Dizziness | 0.3 | Sleepiness | 0.2 |
| Headache | 0.2 | Dry mouth | 0.1 |
| Epigastric pain or cramps | 0.2 | Muscular pain | 0.1 |

TABLE 7. Adverse effects reported by 139/7911 patients (1.76%)

| Type | Patients reporting adverse events | No. adverse events reported | Relationship to "Tagamet"[a] | | | |
|---|---|---|---|---|---|---|
| | | | Related | Questionably related | Not related | Deferred/not shown |
| GI | 61 (0.77%) | 65 | 5 | 43 | 16 | 1 |
| Central nervous system | 30 (0.38%) | 38 | 3 | 27 | 8 | 0 |
| Allergic/Skin | 12 (0.15%) | 13 | 2 | 8 | 3 | 0 |
| Endocrine | 11 (0.14%) | 12 | 5 | 6 | 0 | 1 |
| Musculoskeletal | 6 (0.08%) | 6 | 0 | 4 | 2 | 0 |
| Urinary tract | 6 (0.08%) | 6 | 1 | 2 | 3 | 0 |
| Autonomic | 2 (0.03%) | 2 | 0 | 1 | 1 | 0 |
| Sensory organs | 2 (0.03%) | 2 | 0 | 2 | 0 | 0 |
| Cardiovascular | 6 (0.08%) | 6 | 1 | 1 | 4 | 0 |
| Blood | 1 (0.01%) | 1 | 0 | 0 | 1 | 0 |
| Miscellaneous | 11 (0.14%) | 11 | 1 | 4 | 4 | 2 |
| Total | | 162 | 18 | 98 | 42 | 4 |

[a] As judged by SKF Clinical Monitors.

Once a new drug is in clinical trial or on the market, adverse effects, real or suspected, may be noted which were not predictable from the previous toxicity studies. These may require further, specially designed studies, in either animals or man, to throw more light on the incidence, severity or reality of these adverse effects. The foregoing account of preclinical studies and clinical experience with cimetidine contains examples of both types of studies.

The conventional toxicity studies carried out prior to, and concurrent with, Phase I, II and III studies in man revealed few adverse effects. In view of the occasional reversible granulocytopenia observed in dogs with metiamide, particular attention was paid to the haematological results with cimetidine. No repetition of the effects seen with metiamide occurred and, as indicated above, white cell disorders are extremely uncommon in the clinical use of cimetidine and, even in the rare cases reported, a causal relationship has not been demonstrated unequivocally.

The reduction in size and delay in maturation of secondary sex organs in both rats and dogs in toxicity tests led to studies which established that cimetidine possesses very weak anti-androgenic activity. This is possibly, but not certainly, associated with the occasional reported case of gynaecomastia. The lack of effect of high doses of cimetidine on potency or fertility in reproductive toxicology studies tends to support the current view that cimetidine administration is unlikely to be a cause of impotence.

The statistically significant increase in incidence of benign Leydig cell hyperplasia and tumours seen in both two year rat studies seems to be of no relevance to the clinical use of the drug. The strain of rat used has a high spontaneous incidence of such tumours and experience has shown that chemical insult with high doses of compounds other than cimetidine causes the already high incidence to be increased further.

The cases of mental confusion reported, usually in elderly or severely ill patients, could not have been predicted from the animal tests carried out prior to marketing. Distribution studies using radiolabelled material showed little or no penetration into the central nervous system (Cross, 1977) and behavioural tests with high doses revealed no abnormalities (Brimblecombe and Duncan, 1977). Subsequent studies in man and animals have shown that the drug can penetrate into the cerebro-spinal fluid but in experimental animals the amount reaching brain tissue is very small indeed (Lee, Leslie and Sutton, Personal Communication). The requirement appears to be for an appropriate animal model to predict these effects. As stated above, it is possible that the blood–brain barrier in some patients is compromised. How this could be achieved in animals is not clear and, in any case, it is possible that the behavioural phenomena reported in man would not be reproduced or recognized in lower animals.

The drug interactions now known to occur with cimetidine were not predictable using acute toxicity studies as the test procedure. This type of interaction study is widely demanded by regulatory bodies but the value of the results is not very obvious, especially in view of the very large numbers of animals used. It is noteworthy, for example that the interaction with warfarin did not show up in these tests. The design and interpretation of these studies is a matter for considerable debate and it is almost certain that more complex and more specific tests, e.g. involving preparations of microsomal enzymes, are appropriate for the production of enzyme induction and consequent drug interactions. There would also be a considerable saving in the use of animals.

An example of studies which had to be carried out post-marketing relates to the controversy over whether there is any relationship between cimetidine administration and the development of gastric carcinoma. The only hard evidence on this subject is from the two rat carcinogenicity studies and the long term dog study referred to above. In none of these studies were cancerous or pre-cancerous lesions found in the stomachs of animals treated over long periods of time with high doses of cimetidine.

However, since 1979 there have been anecdotal reports of gastric cancer occurring in patients treated with cimetidine (e.g. Elder *et al.*, 1979). As indicated earlier this, in theory, could be due to the formation of N-nitrosocimetidine or to elevated levels of total N-nitroso compounds due to bacterially-catalysed nitrosation of food-stuffs in the hypochlorhydric stomach. Attempts to throw light on these hypothetical possibilities have led to considerable chemical and biological (*in vitro* and *in vivo* in experimental animals and man) work in our own laboratories and elsewhere. The most likely explanation remains that the gastric carcinomas were present but undiagnosed before cimetidine treatment commenced. Even if N-nitrosocimetidine is formed—and it has not been detected using a method sensitive to concentrations of 50 ng/ml—it would seem unlikely to present a significant hazard since early reports from long-term animal studies suggests a lack of or, at worst, a very low level of carcinogenic activity.

The more general theory of bacterial overgrowth in the hypochlorhydric stomach leading to increased levels of N-nitroso compounds is still under active investigation. On present evidence there is considerable doubt as to whether this occurs in cimetidine treated patients since the pH fluctuates throughout the 24 h period and so bacteria do not permanently colonize the stomach. In any case, much remains to be learned about nitrosation reactions especially at higher pHs. Some of the earlier simplistic views based on inadequate data or limited techniques are almost certainly not correct. Although some of the work has been stimulated by the debate over cimetidine it seems probable that many of the results emerging and the new techniques being developed will be valuable in more general investigations into drug-induced carcinogenesis.

In summary, it can be stated that the animal toxicity studies with cimetidine indicated that it would be, by the standards applied to most drugs, a remarkably safe therapeutic agent. This has been borne out in its clinical use.

# References

Ash, A. S. F. and Schild, H. O. (1966). Receptors mediating some actions of histamine. *Br. J. Pharmacol.* **27**, 427–439.

Bavin, P. M. G., Durant, G. J., Miles, P. D., Mitchell, R. C. and Pepper, E. S. (1980). Nitrosation of cimetidine, [N''-cyano-N-methyl-N''-([2-(5-methyl-imidazol-4-yl)methylthio])ethylguanidine]. *J. Chem. Res. (S)*, 212–213.

Bavin, P. M. G., Darkin, D. W. and Viney, N. J. (1981). Total nitroso compounds in gastric juice. Presented at 7th international meeting on nitroso compounds, I.A.R.C., Tokyo. In Press.

Brimblecombe, R. W. (1980). The toxicology of cimetidine with particular reference to possible nitrosamine formation. Paper presented at the Drug Symposium on Cimetidine, *XI* International Congress on Gastroenterology, Hamburg, June 10.

Brimblecombe, R. W. and Duncan, W. A. M. (1977). The relevance to man of preclinical data for cimetidine. *In* "Cimetidine: Proceedings of the Second International Symposium on Histamine H$_2$-Receptor Antagonists", (Ed. Burland, W. L. and Simkins, M. A.), pp. 54–65. Amsterdam-Oxford: Excerpta Medica.

Brimblecombe, R. W., Duncan, W. A. M., Durant, G. J., Emmett, J. C., Gannellin, C. R., Leslie, G. B. and Parsons, M. E. (1978). Characterisation and development of cimetidine as a histamine H$_2$-receptor antagonist. *Gastroenterology* **74**, 339–347.

Burland, W. L., Gleadle, R. I., Lee, R. M., Rowley-Jones, D. and Groom, G. V. (1979). Prolactin responses to cimetidine. *Br. J. clin. Pharmacol.* **7**, 19–21.

Byron, J. W. (1977). Mechanism for histamine H$_2$-receptor induced cell-cycle changes in the bone marrow stem cell. *Agents and Actions* **7**, 209–213.

Celestin, L. R., Harvey, V., Saunders, J. H. B., Wormsley, K. G., Forrest, J. A. H., Logan, R. F. A., Shearman, D. J. C., Fermont, D., Haggie, S. J., Wyllie, J. H., Albinus, M., Thompson, M. H., Venables, C. W., Burland, W. L., Duncan, W. A. M., Hawkins, B. W. and Sharpe, P. C. (1975). Treatment of duodenal ulcer by metiamide. A multicentre trial. *Lancet* **ii**, 779–781.

Colin-Jones, D., Langman, M. J. S., Lawson, D. H. and Vessey, M. P. (1981). Postmarketing surveillance. *In* "Cimetidine in the 1980s", (Ed. Brown, J. H.), pp. 270–274. Edinburgh: Churchill Livingstone.

Crean, G. P., Morson, B. C., Leslie, G. B. and Roe, F. J. C. (1981a). Cimetidine: Further evidence of noncarcinogenicity in dogs. *New Engl. J. Med.* **304** (11), 672.

Crean, G. P., Leslie, G. B., Walker, T. F., Whitehead, S. M. and Roe, F. J. C. (1981b). Safety evaluation of cimetidine: 54 month interim report on long-term study in dogs. *J. Appl. Toxicol.* **1**, 159–164.

Cross, S. A. M. (1977). The localisation of metiamide and cimetidine using autoradiographical techniques. *In* "Proceedings, 18th Meeting of the European Society of Toxicology, Edinburgh", 1976, vol. 18, (Ed. Duncan, W. A. M. and Leonard, B. J.), pp. 288–290. Amsterdam-Oxford: Excerpta Medica.

Davis, T. G., Pickett, D. L. and Schlosser, J. H. (1980). Evaluation of a worldwide spontaneous reporting system with cimetidine. *J. Am. med. Ass.* **243**, 1912–1914.

Eisenbrand, G. (1981). Discussion Section in Gastric cancer: endogenous factors (Banbury Report 7), (Ed. Bruce, W. R. *et al.*), pp. 445–6 Cold Spring Harbor Laboratory.

Elder, J. B., Ganguli, P. C. and Gillespie, I. E. (1979). Cimetidine and gastric cancer. *Lancet* i, 1005–1006.

Enzmann, G. D., Leonard, J. M., Paulsen, C. A. and Rogers, J. (1981). Effect of cimetidine on reproductive function in men. *Clin. Res.* **29**, 26A.

Finney, D. J. (1971). "Prohibit Analysis". 3rd Edition Cambridge University Press. 230–268.

Flind, A. C., Rowley-Jones, D. and Backhouse, J. N. (1980). The safety of cimetidine: a continuing assessment. *In* "$H_2$-receptor Antagonists", Proc. Eur. Symposium, Capri, October 18–20, 1979, (Ed. Torsoli, A. *et al.*), pp. 209–217. Amsterdam, Oxford: Excerpta Medica.

Flind, A. C. and Rowley-Jones, D. (1982). The endocrinological effects of cimetidine. "Japanese Tagamet Symposium". In Press.

Forrest, J. A. H., Shearman, D. J. C., Spence, R. and Celestin, L. R. (1975). Neutropenia associated with metiamide. *Lancet*, i, 392–393.

Foster, A. B., Jarman, M., Manson, D. and Schulten, H. R. (1980). Structure and reactivity of nitrosocimetidine. *Cancer Lett.* **9**, 47–52.

Ghosh, M. N. and Schild, H. O. (1958). Continuous recording of acid gastric secretion in the rat. *Br. J. Pharmacol.* **13**, 54–61.

Gifford, L. M., Aeugle, M. E., Myerson, R. M. and Tannenbaum, P. J. (1980). Results of the Tagamet post-market surveillance program in the United States. *In* "Second National Symposium on Cimetidine, Brussels", 1979, (Ed. Dresse, A. L. *et al.*), pp. 89–105. Amsterdam, Oxford: Excerpta Medica.

Gombar, C. T., Jensen, D. E. and Magee, P. N. (1981). Methylation of DNA *in vivo* by the nitroso-derivative of cimetidine. *Proc Am. Ass. Cancer Res.* **22**, 81 abstr. 320.

Griffiths, R., Lee, R. M. and Taylor, D. C. (1977). Kinetics of cimetidine in man and experimental animals. *In* "Cimetidine: Proceedings of the Second International Symposium on Histamine $H_2$-Receptor Antagonists", (ed. Burland, W. L. and Simkins, M. A.), pp. 38–51. Amsterdam-Oxford: Excerpta Medica.

Hisaw, F. L. (1959). Comparative effectiveness of estrogens on fluid imbibition and growth of the rat's uterus. *Endocrinology* **64**, 276–289.

Illingworth, R. N. and Jarvie, D. R. (1979). Absence of toxicity in cimetidine overdosage. *Br. Med. J.* **1**, 453–454.

Jensen, D. E. and Magee, P. N. (1981). Methylation of DNA by nitrosocimetidine *in vitro*. *Cancer Res.* **41**, 230–236.

Jost, A. (1947). Sex differentiation in rabbit embryos. *Archs. Anat. microsc. Morphol. exp.* **36**, 242–270.

Leslie, G. B. and Walker, T. F. (1977). A toxicological profile of cimetidine. *In* "Cimetidine: Proceedings of the Second International Symposium on Histamine $H_2$-Receptor Antagonists", (ed. Burland, W. L. and Simkins, M. A.), pp. 24–33. Amsterdam-Oxford: Excerpta Medica.

Leslie, G. B., Noakes, D. N., Pollitt, F. D., Roe, F. J. C. and Walker, T. F. (1981). A two-year study with cimetidine in the rat: assessment for chronic toxicity and carcinogenicity. *Toxicol. Appl. Pharmacol.* **61**, 119–137.

Litchfield, J. T. and Wilcoxon, F. (1949). A simplified method of evaluating dose–effect experiments. *J. Pharmacol. exp. Ther.* **96**, 99-113.

Milton-Thompson, G. J., Lightfoot, N. F., Ahmet, Z., Hunt, R. H., Barnard, J., Bavin, P. M. G., Brimblecombe, R. W., Darkin, D. W., Moore, P. J. and Viney, N. (1982). Intragastric acidity bacteria, nitrite and N-nitrosocompounds before, during and after cimetidine treatment. *Lancet.* In press.

Neuvonen, P. J., Tokola, R. A. and Kaste, M. (1980). Cimetidine-phenytoin interaction: effect on serum phenytoin concentration and antipyrine test in man. *Naunyn-Schmiedebergs Arch.* **313** (Supplement) R60.

Neumann, F., Richter, K. D. and Guenzel, P. (1965). Wirkungen von antiandrogenen. *Z. Vet.-med.* A, **12**, 171–178.

Parsons, M. E. (1969). Quantitative studies of drug-induced acid gastric secretion. Ph.D thesis, University of London.

Pool, B. L., Eisenbrand, G. and Schmahl, D. (1979). Biological activity of nitrosated cimetidine. *Toxicology* **15**, 69–72.

Reed, P. I., Haines, K., Smith, P. L. R., House, F. R. and Walters, C. L. (1981). Effect of cimetidine on gastric juice N-nitrosamine concentration. *Lancet* **ii**, 553–556.

Rowley-Jones, D. and Flind, A. C. (1981). Continuing evaluation of the safety of cimetidine. *In* "Cimetidine in the 1980s", (Ed. Baron, J. H.), pp. 261–269. Edinburgh: Churchill Livingstone.

Schoental, R. (1966). Carcinogenic activity of N-methyl-N-nitroso-N'-nitroguanidine. *Nature* **209**, 726–727.

Serlin, M. J., Sibeon, R. G., Mossman, S., Breckenridge, A. M., Williams, J. R. B., Atwood, J. L. and Willoughby, J. M. T. (1979). Cimetidine: interaction with oral anticoagulants in man. *Lancet* **ii**, 317–319.

Sharpe, P. C. and Hawkins, B. W. (1977). Efficacy and safety of cimetidine. Long term treatment with cimetidine. *In* "Cimetidine: Proceedings of the Second International Symposium on Histamine $H_2$-Receptor Antagonists", (Ed. Burland, W. L. and Simkins, M. A.), pp. 358–366. Amsterdam-Oxford: Excerpta Medica.

Sivelle, P. C., Underwood, A. H. and Jelly, J. A. (1982). The effects of histamine $H_2$-receptor antagonists on androgen actions *in vivo* and dihydrotestosterone binding to the rat prostate androgen receptor *in vitro*. *Biochem. Pharmacol.* **31**, 677–684.

Sugimura, T. and Fujimura, S. (1967). Tumour production in glandular stomachs of rat by N-methyl-N'-nitro-N-nitrosoguanidine. *Nature*, **216**, 943–944.

Taylor, D. C., Creswell, P. R. and Bartlett, D. C. (1978). The metabolism and elimination of cimetidine, a histamine $H_2$-receptor antagonist, in the rat, dog and man. *Drg. Metab. Dispos.* **6**, 21–30.

Van Thiel, D. H., Gavaler, J. S., Smith, W. I. and Paul, G. (1979). Hypothalamic-pituitary-gonadal dysfunction in men using cimetidine. *New Engl. J. Med.* **300**, 1012–1015.

Whitehead, S. M. and Leslie, G. B. (1983). Endoscopic Examination of Cimetidine-treated Dogs *In* "Situation Actuelle et Orientations Futures en Toxicologie du Medicament". John Libbey Eurotext: Paris and London 234–235.

Wiesner, B. P. (1934). The post-natal development of the genital organs in the Albino rat. With a discussion of a new theory of sexual differentiation. *J. Obstet Gynae. Br. Commonw.* **41**, 867–922.

Wyllie, J. H., Hesselbo, T. and Black, J. W. (1972). Effects in man of histamine $H_2$-receptor blockade by burimamide. *Lancet* **ii**, 1117–1120.

# 5

# Beta-adrenoceptor blocking drugs: pronethalol, propranolol and practolol

J. M. CRUICKSHANK, J. D. FITZGERALD and M. TUCKER

*ICI PLC, Pharmaceuticals Division, Alderley Park,*
*Macclesfield, Cheshire, England*

## I. Summary

Beta-adrenoceptor antagonists now comprise a large group of agents which are administered to patients world-wide, chiefly for the management of hypertension and symptomatic coronary artery disease (angina pectoris and myocardial infarction). The first beta antagonists to be administered to man for these clinical indications were pronethalol and propranolol, which were discovered and developed in the ICI laboratories between 1960 and 1964.

In chronic toxicity studies pronethalol was well tolerated in rats (250 mg/kg) and dogs (150 mg/kg) except for occasional central nervous system manifestations. In three oncogenicity studies in mice, pronethalol was shown to increase the incidence of thymic lymphosarcomata. No carcinogenic effect was observed in subsequent studies in rats, guinea pigs, dogs and monkeys, but pronethalol was withdrawn from clinical use. Propranolol is a more potent and specific beta antagonist than pronethalol. Given orally to rats (200 mg/kg) and dogs (125 mg/kg), propranolol caused collapse (rats) and severe vomiting (dogs). However, in clinical doses it is well tolerated. No teratogenic or oncogenic effects were observed.

Practolol, the first $\beta_1$ selective antagonist, was much better tolerated than pronethalol or propranolol in higher doses, given either acutely or chronically. In a 13 week rat study, practolol in the highest dose (500 mg/kg), caused bladder epithelial hyperplasia in rats, which was reversible. This was attributed to a local irritant effect due to transient peak urinary concentrations of practolol associated with daily oral dosing. When practolol was given in 1,000 mg/kg *in the diet*, bladder hyperplasia was not observed. No abnormalities were detected in dogs or in the prolonged oncogenicity studies in mice and rats. Practolol given in a 10% solution to rabbit eyes caused no changes.

The unwanted effects of beta antagonists in man comprise those due either to the consequences of their pharmacological actions or to a non-specific effect. Unwanted effects such as bradycardia, hypotension, heart failure, bronchial spasm, cold extremities and easy fatiguability are attributable to the known actions of beta antagonists. With the exception of bradycardia, none of these were predicted from the initial animal studies. A variety of side effects not clearly attributable to specific beta blockade have been reported with propranolol. Complaints of vivid dreams, light-headedness, dizziness and ill-defined central nervous system effects are associated with propranolol administration. Other effects include vomiting, diarrhoea, and skin rashes.

Practolol appeared to be the best tolerated beta antagonist in both the initial animal toxicity studies and the subsequent clinical evaluation. However, the unique oculomucocutaneous syndrome, which was first observed four years after marketing, led to the withdrawal of practolol, except for short term administration. This syndrome cannot be reproduced in any of the animal species studied and its aetiology remains unexplained. It is a classic example of the failure of prolonged animal toxicity testing to predict a serious unwanted effect in man.

## II. Introduction

The subdivision of postsynaptic adrenoceptors into alpha and beta was suggested by Ahlquist in 1948 (Ahlquist, 1948). This subdivision was based on the differences in efficacy of a series of catecholamines when examined for their effects on a variety of smooth muscle preparations. This hypothesis explained the dual and often opposing effects of adrenaline observed by Dale in the presence of ergot (Dale, 1906). Ergot, and subsequently phenoxybenzamine and dibenzyline, were shown to antagonize the vasoconstrictor actions of noradrenaline and adrenaline. Such an effect, according to the Ahlquist hypothesis, is termed alpha adrenoceptor antagonism. The most specific agonist at beta adrenoceptors is isoprenaline (isoproterenol) but no specific beta antagonist was available until ten years after Alquist's publication.

Powell and Slater (1958) studied a series of analogues of isoprenaline in the search for a long acting bronchodilator drug and observed that the dichloro analogue (DCI) antagonized rather than mimicked the action of isoprenaline on tracheal smooth muscle. Moran and Perkins (1958) showed that DCI was a specific antagonist at beta adrenoceptors and introduced the term "beta antagonist".

In 1958, Dr. J. W. Black joined ICI Pharmaceuticals Division and instituted the programme of research designed to discover a beta antagonist of higher potency and specificity than DCI, without its marked beta stimulant (partial agonist or intrinsic sympathomimetic) activity. It must be appreciated that this was designed drug discovery, the purpose of which was to find a novel therapy for the treatment of myocardial ischaemia (i.e., both angina pectoris and acute myocardial infarction). Black (1967) subsequently wrote: "We hoped that beta adrenergic blockade would reduce the consumption of oxygen by the ischaemic myocardium and thus have the same net effect as increasing its oxygen supply. The possibility that the treatment of patients with myocardial ischaemia, with or without an actual infarction, with adrenergic beta receptor antagonists might prolong lives was part of our speculations about the therapeutic use of these drugs".

This novel conceptual approach distinguishes his work from that of both Powell and Slater (1958), with DCI, and Lish *et al.* with sotalol (1965), both of whom discovered beta antagonists whilst looking for beta stimulants for use in bronchial asthma. DCI was studied in man, but only for its effects on arrhythmias associated with phaeochromocytoma (a rare catecholamine secreting tumour) (Riddell *et al.*, 1963).

Pronethalol was discovered in March 1960 and by December 1962 was shown to increase exercise tolerance when given in a single oral dose to patients with angina pectoris (Dornhorst and Robinson, 1962). Prolonged toxicity studies showed that pronethalol produced thymic tumours in the Alderley Park strain of mice, and it was withdrawn from clinical use (Tucker, 1968).

Propranolol was discovered in 1962 and introduced into clinical usage in 1965. It is the reference beta antagonist. Propranolol causes specific competitive antagonism at the beta adrenoceptor site and this is the hallmark of this class of agent (Barrett and Fitzgerald, 1968). Beta antagonists developed after propranolol may differ pharmacologically from it in certain respects. These are: (1) The presence and degree of partial agonist activity (PAA) or intrinsic activity. (2) The relative affinity for either $\beta_1$ or $\beta_2$ adrenoceptors (i.e. selectivity). (3) The presence of membrane stabilizing activity (MSA) which is related to the physicochemical nature of the compound, i.e. lipophilicity (Cruickshank, 1981). (4) Inhibitory effects at alpha adrenoceptors (e.g. labetalol) or on non-adrenoceptor smooth muscle tonic mechanisms, (e.g. prizidolol) (Fitzgerald, 1969, 1982).

This chapter will be confined to a description of the toxicological studies performed on the first three beta antagonists developed by ICI, namely pronethalol, propranolol and practolol. Pronethalol was the first beta antagonist in which a beneficial effect in angina pectoris was demonstrated (Dornhorst and Robinson, 1962). It differs from propranolol in being only one tenth as potent and having significant partial agonist activity. Practolol differs from propranolol in being relatively selective for the $\beta_1$ adrenoceptor as well as possessing modest partial agonist activity and no membrane stabilizing properties. In high doses in animals, practolol was better tolerated than either pronethalol or propranolol. It was effective as an anti-anginal and anti-hypertensive agent and was well tolerated (Wiseman, 1971). In 1974/5 the unique oculomucocutaneous syndrome was associated with practolol administration. This syndrome comprises psoriasiform rash, keratoconjunctivitis, secretory otitis media and a sclerosing fibrosis of the endothelial lining of the pericardial, plural and peritoneal cavities.

These pathological changes have not been detected in a variety of other species and, considering the extent of the usage of practolol, the syndrome occurs in relatively few patients. If the incidence was similar in a susceptible animal species, then very large numbers would need to be studied to detect an effect. The cause is unknown, and practolol has been withdrawn from clinical use, except for parenteral administration for the control of life-threatening arrhythmias. In the following sections, the animal and human toxicology of these three agents is summarized from the point of view of the predictive value of animal data as a guide to novel agents for human use.

## III. Preclinical studies

The preclinical toxicology studies which are reported here only include those studies carried out before marketing. All of the studies were performed between 1960 and 1971, and by present day standards for toxicology studies, the number of animals used was small and the duration of treatment short; kinetic and metabolic studies, in particular, were limited. After propranolol and practolol were marketed many additional studies were carried out to update the toxicology to modern standards and to expand greatly kinetic and metabolic work in animals and man. These studies are not reported here, but the results of these additional studies did not produce any finding which had not been observed in the original studies.

## A. Pronethalol ("Alderlin")

Preclinical studies with pronethalol are shown in Table 1. The studies were all carried out between 1960 and 1963.

1. Results

*(a) Acute Toxicity Tests*
The oral $LD_{50}$ was 800 mg/kg (mice) and 1000 mg/kg (rats). Deaths after

TABLE 1. Preclinical studies with pronethalol

| Type of study | Species | Number | Dose (mg/kg) | Duration |
|---|---|---|---|---|
| Acute tests | Rat | 5/group | Various | 1 week |
| | Mouse | 10/group | Various | 1 week |
| | Monkey | 2♂2♀ | 200 mg/kg | 1 day |
| Chronic tests | Rat | 25/sex/group | 0. 40, 100, 250 po | 12 weeks |
| | Rat | 20/sex/group | 0, 50, 100, 200 po | 52 weeks |
| | Dog | 1/sex/group | 0, 40, 150 po | 4 weeks |
| | Dog | 4/sex  8/sex | 0,  125 po } | 26 weeks |
| | Monkey | 2/sex/group | 0, 100 po | 52 weeks |
| Teratogenic tests | Mouse | 30♀/group | 0, 0.2% diet | Throughout |
| | Rat | 20♀/group | 0, 0.2% diet | |
| | Rabbit | 10♀ | 0 | pregnancy |
| | | 13♀ | 0.2%/diet | |
| Oncogenicity tests | Mouse | 46/sex | 0 | 52 weeks |
| | | 56/sex | 20 p.o. | |
| | Mouse | 25/sex/group | 0, 50, 100, 200 po | 41 weeks |
| | Mouse | 25/sex/group | 0, 50, 100, 200 in diet | 41 weeks |

oral doses all occurred within 24 h of dosing. The intravenous $LD_{50}$ was 40 mg/kg (mice) and 45 mg/kg (rats). Deaths after intravenous dosing occurred within five minutes. No effects were seen in rhesus monkeys given a single oral dose of 200 mg/kg.

### (b) Chronic Toxicity Tests

*(i) Rats* No treatment-related effects were seen in rats treated for four weeks with daily oral doses up to 250 mg/kg. In the 52 week study, mortality was increased in all the treated groups; four of the animals which died were observed to have attacks of dyspnoea and bradycardia shortly after dosing and two were dosed with atropine which produced a rapid return of normal heart and respiration rates. It was considered that the deaths may have been related to inhalation of dosing fluid; to prevent regurgitation of doses the route of administration was changed to subcutaneous administration. The compound proved to be very irritant by this route and thereafter the drug was incorporated into the diet. Weight gains were similar in treated and control groups, there were no effects on plasma potassium levels or any changes in haematological examinations. No histological changes attributable to pronethalol were seen in any animal which died during the study or in any which were killed after 52 weeks treatment.

*(ii) Dogs* In the four week dog study animals dosed at 150 mg/kg, after overnight fasting, showed subdued behaviour, incoordination and convul-

sions shortly after dosing; these signs resolved within 6 h of dosing and when the animals were dosed 1 h after feeding no further toxic signs were observed. No treatment-related effects were seen in body weights, or haematological or biochemical examinations, and there were no pathological changes attributable to pronethalol. The dogs treated for 52 weeks were dosed after feeding but clinical signs of toxicity, similar to those seen in the four week study, were observed sporadically in treated animals and one female died in convulsions in the sixth week. There were no other changes attributable to pronethalol in body weights, or haematological, biochemical and urine examinations, which were made at regular intervals throughout the study. All animals were necropsied and there were no histological changes related to treatment.

### (c) Teratogenicity Tests

All animals in the teratogenic tests were fed a diet containing 0.2% pronethalol throughout pregnancy. The rats and mice were allowed to litter normally and raise their offspring to weaning. Rabbits were killed on day 28 of pregnancy and the foetuses removed and radiographed. No teratogenic effects were observed in these three species.

### (d) Oncogenicity Tests

The first oncogenicity study in mice had a high mortality in both control and treated animals which was attributed, chiefly, to aspiration of dosing fluid. No clinical signs relating to treatment were seen during the study and weight gains were similar in control and treated groups. All animals, whether dying or surviving to the end of the study, were given a full necropsy and histological examination. The results indicated an increase in thymic lymphosarcomata in the dosed group and two further studies were done to confirm this. The incidence of tumours in all three studies is given in Table 2 and these results were published by Paget (1963).

The results of these studies indicated that pronethalol had a potential carcinogenic effect in the Alderley Park strain of mouse and the compound was withdrawn from further development. Subsequently many further long term tests were made in mice, rats, guinea pigs, dogs and monkeys (Alcock and Bond, 1964) but no carcinogenic effect was observed in any species other than the mouse (Alderley Park strain).

It was postulated by Rose and Howe (personal communication) that the carcinogenicity of pronethalol could be due to the formation of an ethyleneimine from the side chain of pronethalol; such a metabolite would be highly reactive and unlikely to be detectable as a metabolite. They suggested that the corresponding betachloroethylamine (ICI 42,464) which does not possess beta blocking activity, would give rise to an ethyleneimine *in vivo* and this compound was tested for any carcinogenic effect in rats and

TABLE 2. Incidence of tumours in mice treated with pronethalol

| Test No | Dose | Number of mice | No. and type of tumour |
|---------|------|----------------|------------------------|
| 1 | Control | 92 | 3 thymic lymphosarcomas |
| | 200 mg/kg | 104 | 14 thymic lymphosarcomas 2 lung adenomas |
| 2 | Control | 50 | 1 thymic lymphosarcoma |
| | 50 mg/kg | 50 | 1 thymic lymphosarcoma |
| | 100 mg/kg | 50 | 2 thymic lymphosarcomas 2 reticulum cell sarcomas |
| | 200 mg/kg | 50 | 2 thymic lymphosarcomas |
| 3 | Control | 50 | 1 adenocarcinoma salivary gland |
| | 0.05% diet | 50 | 3 thymic lymphosarcomas |
| | 0.1% diet | 50 | 5 thymic lymphosarcomas |
| | 0.2% diet | 50 | 6 thymic lymphosarcomas 1 lung adenoma 2 reticulum cell sarcomas |

mice. The results (Tucker, 1968) indicated that ICI 42,464 was a potent carcinogen in both species, producing thymic lymphosarcomata in mice and mammary carcinomas and leukaemias in rats. Pronethalol was not carcinogenic in the rat and the existence of an ethyleneimine as a metabolite in the mouse is hypothetical since it was not demonstrated to be present.

Other workers have tested pronethalol for carcinogenic effects. Murmann (personal communication) and Newberne et al. (1977) failed to demonstrate a carcinogenic effect with pronethalol in several strains of mice. Thymic lymphosarcomata in the mouse have been attributed to the presence of oncogenic viruses within a colony and one theory for the different results obtained in experiments at ICI and other laboratories is the presence of such viruses in some of the colonies and their absence in others.

*(e) Metabolism*

A method of analysis for pronethalol in blood was not available at the time of the preclinical studies. Limited metabolic studies were made in four species—rat, mouse, rabbit and guinea pig. Three main groups of metabolites were identified in the urine; in the rat and rabbit equal amounts of acidic basic and neutral exponents were excreted; in the guinea pig 66–70% was excreted as an acidic metabolite and in the mouse excretion was almost entirely of neutral components.

# B. Propranolol ("Inderal")

Toxicity studies with propranolol are shown in Table 3. The studies were all carried out between 1963 and 1966.

TABLE 3. Preclinical studies with propranolol

| Type of study | Species | Number | Dose (mg/kg) | Duration |
|---|---|---|---|---|
| Acute tests | Rat | 5/group | Various | 2 weeks |
| | Mouse | 10/group | Various | 2 weeks |
| | Rabbit | 1/group | Various | 2 weeks |
| | Monkey | ♂1♀ | 1–6 mg/kg iv | 2 weeks |
| Chronic tests | Rat | 10/sex/group | 0, 50, 200 po | 13 weeks |
| | Rat | 25/sex/group | 0, 5, 50, 150 po | 78 weeks |
| | Mouse | 10/sex/group | 0, 50, 200 po | 13 weeks |
| | Dog | 3/sex/group | 0, 20, 60 po | 13 weeks |
| | Dog | 4/sex/group | 0, 5, 20, 60 po | 52 weeks |
| Teratogenic tests | Rat 1 | 10♀ | 200 | Days 6–20 pregnancy |
| | Rat 2 | 10♀/group | 0, 5, 50, 150 po | Pregnancy, lactation |
| | Rat 3 | 10♀/group | 0.005, 0.05, 0.15% diet | Pregnancy, lactation |
| | Rat 4 | 12♀/group | 0.005, 0.05% diet | Days 6–20 pregnancy |
| | Rat 5 | 15♀/group | 0.005, 0.05% diet | Pregnancy, lactation |
| | Rat 6 | 24/sex/group | 0, 0.005, 0.05% diet | 2 pregnancies |
| | Rabbit | 12♀/group | 0, 0.0125, 0.125, 0.25% diet | Pregnancy, lactation |
| Ocular toxicity | Rabbit | 3/group | 0.1%, 1.0% | 4 × daily–2 weeks |
| Oncogenicity test | Mouse | 30/sex/group | 0, 150 po | 80 weeks |

## 1. Results

### (a) Acute Toxicity Tests

The $LD_{50}$ after oral administration was 500 mg/kg (rabbits), 500 mg/kg (mice) and 1000 mg/kg (rats). The intravenous $LD_{50}$ was >7.5 mg/kg (rabbits), 30 mg/kg (mice) and 25 mg/kg (rats). Animals which died after ·intravenous dosing did so within 1 h: deaths after oral dosing occurred within 24 h, some in convulsion, others with a slow respiration rate and incoordination. The maximum tolerated intravenous dose in monkeys was 6 mg/kg.

### (b) Chronic Toxicity Tests

(i) Rats In a 13 week study animals receiving the highest dose (200 mg/kg/day) did not gain weight at the same rate as the controls and there were several deaths, shortly after dosing, which were attributed to acute toxic effects. Haematological and urine examinations did not show any treatment-related effects. All animals were necropsied and tissues taken for examination; there were no histological changes related to propranolol treatment.

In the 78 week study in rats the compound was administered by catheter for the first six months and then in the diet. Mortality during the study is shown in Table 4. The larger number of deaths at the highest dose during the first six months were due to the acute toxic effects of propranolol at this high dose. Pathological changes in these animals included pulmonary congestion and dilatation of the heart. The increase in deaths in all groups in the final stages of the study were due to an intercurrent infection wtih *Pasteurella pneumotropica;* all animals surviving to this time were treated with chlortetracycline for the final four months of the study. Blood samples (for haematology) and urine samples were taken from control and highest dose groups at

TABLE 4. Mortality rates in 78 week study with propranolol in rats (25/group)

| Time (months) | Control | Males 5 mg/kg | 50 mg/kg | 150 mg/kg | Control | Females 5 mg/kg | 50 mg/kg | 150 mg/kg |
|---|---|---|---|---|---|---|---|---|
| 0–3 | 2 | 1 | 0 | 3 | 0 | 0 | 1 | 9 |
| 4–6 | 0 | 0 | 2 | 3 | 1 | 0 | 1 | 2 |
| 7–9 | 0 | 0 | 3 | 2 | 0 | 1 | 2 | 1 |
| 10–12 | 0 | 0 | 1 | 1 | 3 | 1 | 0 | 1 |
| 13–15 | 2 | 4 | 5 | 3 | 2 | 1 | 2 | 3 |
| 16–18 | 2 | 3 | 2 | 3 | 2 | 0 | 0 | 2 |
| Survived to end | 19 | 17 | 12 | 10 | 17 | 22 | 19 | 7 |

TABLE 5. Incidence of heart lesions in rats treated with propranolol for 78 weeks

| Histological change | Dose group (25/group) | | | |
| --- | --- | --- | --- | --- |
| | 0 | 5 mg/kg | 50 mg/kg | 150 mg/kg |
| Dilated heart | 5 | 7 | 4 | 14 |
| Myocarditis | 3 | 16 | 13 | 11 |

three monthly intervals. No treatment-related changes were observed. Heart rates were measured in all surviving animals immediately prior to necropsy. A reduced heart rate, related to the pharmacological effect of the compound, was seen at the two lower doses but not at the highest dose. No significant differences from controls were seen in the weight of major organs in animals surviving to the end of the study. All animals were necropsied and examined histologically. The incidence of tumours was similar in all groups. Histological changes related to propranolol were found in the heart and these are shown in Table 5. The incidence of chronic myocarditis was increased but the degree was not severe in any animal; in most it consisted of one to several microscopical foci of inflammatory cells with necrosis of single myocytes.

*(ii) Mice* Mice in the 13 week study showed clinical signs, at the highest dose (200 mg/kg), similar to those seen in the rat; there were a few deaths occurring shortly after dosing, and weight gains were less rapid in both dosed groups compared with controls. Haematological examinations did not show any treatment-related effects nor were there any histological changes related to treatment.

*(iii) Dogs* In the 13 week study dosing commenced at 50 and 125 mg/kg/ day after overnight fasting; at these dose levels the compound produced severe vomiting and dosing ceased for several days: the compound was thereafter administered 2 h after feeding and the doses were reduced to 20 and 60 mg/kg/dog for 12 weeks. After the dose level was reduced weight gains were similar in all groups; no treatment-related effects were seen in the haematological, biochemical or urine examinations which were done at intervals throughout the study. All animals were necropsied, the major organs weighed and tissues sampled for histological examination. There were no histological changes related to treatment.

In the 52 week study in dogs, all animals were in good condition through-out the study with similar weights gains in all groups. Samples for haematology, biochemistry and urine samples were taken at three monthly intervals and there were no treatment-related changes. All animals were necropsied and major organs weighed. All treated animals showed a slight increase in the weight of the heart when expressed as a percentage of body weight. The only histological change attributable to propranolol was seen at the highest dose only, consisting of slight oedema and irregularity of glands in the mucosa of the gastric fundus.

### (c) Teratogenic Tests

In all of the teratogenic studies, half of the pregnant animals were killed the day prior to normal parturition and the foetuses removed, stained with alizarin and examined for skeletal abnormalities; the remaining females were allowed to litter normally and rear the young to weaning.

There were six teratogenic studies in the rat. The first study was limited to ten female rats dosed with 200 mg/kg of propranalol from days 6 to 20 of pregnancy. No teratogenic effects were observed. Two more studies followed, with groups receiving various dose levels, between 5 and 150 mg/kg, of propranolol. These doses were administered throughout pregnancy and lactation, by catheter in the second study and diet in the third study. No teratogenic effects were observed but in both studies there was an increase in neonatal deaths in treated animals. Two further studies were done to investigate this effect with propranalol administered in the diet. There were no teratogenic effects or any increase in neonatal deaths. The sixth study included animals dosed with propranolol continuously through mating, pregnancy and lactation for two pregnancies. There were no treatment-related effects. The teratogenic study in the rabbit did not demonstrate any teratogenic effect.

### (d) Ocular Toxicity

The rabbits in this study received instillations of 10% solutions into the eye four times daily for two weeks. Observations and opthalmoscopic examinations were made daily by two independent observers. No changes were seen in the eyes.

### (e) Oncogenic Study

In the 80 week study in mice the dose was administered by catheter for 44 weeks and thereafter in the diet. There was no difference in tumour incidence between treated and control animals.

### (f) Pharmacokinetics and Metabolism

Blood levels of propranolol were determined in the 78 week study in rats in the highest dose group only. The results demonstrated that accumulation occurred at the high level after repeated oral administration but a constant level was achieved by 13 weeks. The mean peak level achieved over the first six months after dosing by catheter was 6 $\mu$g/ml; after 12 months dietary administration peak levels were slightly lower.

More extensive studies were made in the 13 week and the 52 week study in dogs (after 2, 14, 26, 40 and 50 weeks) at all dose levels. The peak levels achieved in both studies were 1.1 $\mu$g/ml at 60 mg/kg, 0.5 $\mu$g/ml at 20 mg/kg and 0.086 $\mu$g/ml at 5 mg/kg. There were no sex differences in blood levels, no obvious accumulation after prolonged dosing and a dose response was apparent. When propranolol was dosed orally to rat, mouse, guinea pig and rabbit at 2 mg/kg, none of the unchanged compound could be detected in the urine or faeces. Metabolic studies with $^{14}$C propranolol were made in the rat where 90% of the radioactivity recovered was found in the urine during the first three days of dosing.

## C. Practolol ("Eraldin")

Toxicity studies with practolol are shown in Table 6. The studies were all carried out between 1967 and 1971.

TABLE 6. Preclinical studies with practolol

| Type of study | Species | Number | Dose (mg/kg) | Duration |
|---|---|---|---|---|
| Acute tests | Mouse | 10/sex/group | Various | 1 week |
| | Rats | 5/sex/group | Various | 1 week |
| | Rabbits | 2/sex/group | Various | 1 week |
| | Monkeys | 3♂3♀ | 1–25 mg/kg po | 2 weeks |
| Chronic tests | Rat | 10/sex/group | 0, 20, 100, 500 po | 13 weeks |
| | Rat | 10♂/group | 0, 1.0% diet | 13 weeks |
| | Dog | 4/sex/group | 0, 10, 50, 200 po | 13 weeks |
| | Dog | 7/sex/group | 0, 10, 50, 200 po | 52 weeks |
| | Dog | 1/sex | 0 | |
| | | 2/sex | 10 mg/kg iv | 4 weeks |
| Teratogenic tests | Rat | 15♀/group | 0, 20, 100, 500 po | Days 6–15 pregnancy |
| | Rabbit | 13♀/group | 0, 50, 100, 250 po | Days 6–28 pregnancy |
| Ocular toxicity | Rabbit | 2 | 10% solution | 1 day |
| | Rabbit | 6 | 10% solution | 3 × daily–3 weeks |
| Oncogenicity tests | Mouse | 25/sex/group | 0, 20, 100 po | 80 weeks |
| | Rat | 20/sex/group | 0, 0.04, 0.2% diet | 104 weeks |

1. Results

*(a) Acute Toxicity Tests*

Oral $LD_{50}$s were not found since doses of 2000 mg/kg in rats and mice and 1000  mg/kg in rabbits did not produce any effects. The intravenous $LD_{50}$ for mice was between 100 and 110 mg/kg, for rats 84 mg/kg and for rabbits between 50 and 75 mg/kg. Deaths after intravenous dosing occurred within a few seconds of dosing and no clinical signs were observed in survivors at any dose 1 h after dosing. No clinical effects were seen in rhesus monkeys given seven daily intravenous doses rising from 1 to 25 mg/kg. Blood samples, for haematology and clinical chemistry, and urine samples were taken from the monkeys after 7 days; no treatment-related changes were observed and necropsies and histological examinations did not show any treatment-related effects.

*(b) Chronic Toxicity Tests*

*(i) Rats* In the 13 week study in rats, two animals, one in each of the low and middle dose groups, died after aspiration of dosing fluid. Male rats at the highest dose failed to gain weight as rapidly as controls during the final six weeks. Blood samples, for haematology and clinical chemistry, and urine samples were examined at regular intervals and no treatment-related effects were observed. The major organs were weighed at necropsy and there were no significant differences from controls. All animals received a full necropsy and histological examination. The only histological change attributable to practolol was hyperplasia of the transitional cell epithelium of the urinary bladder at the highest dose. The incidence is shown in Table 7. The

TABLE 7. Incidence of bladder epithelial hyperplasia in rats treated with practolol for 13 weeks

| | | Dose | | |
| Degree of hyperplasia | Control N = 20 | 20 mg/kg 20 | 100 mg/kg 20 | 500 mg/kg 20 |
|---|---|---|---|---|
| Normal (1–2 cells thick) | 15 | 16 | 14 | 7 |
| Grade 1 hyperplasia (2–3 cells thick) | 4 | 4 | 5 | 2 |
| Grade 2 hyperplasia (3–4 cells thick) | 1 | 0 | 0 | 5 |
| Grade 3 hyperplasia (4–5 cells thick) | 0 | 0 | 0 | 4 |
| Grade 4 hyperplasia (5–6 cells thick) | 0 | 0 | 0 | 2 |

hyperplasia was not accompanied by any other change. Ten rats which had been dosed in parallel with the highest dose for 13 weeks were left undosed for a further four weeks and the animals were then killed and the bladders taken for histological examination. There was no bladder epithelial hyperplasia in these animals. It was considered that the very large dose of practolol (500 mg/kg/day) could have given rise to high concentrations of the compound in the urine, since more than 90% was excreted in the urine in the rat, and this might have had a local irritant effect. If high concentrations were avoided this local effect would not occur. To prove this, a second 13 week study in rats was undertaken consisting of ten control males and ten dosed males fed a diet containing practolol at a concentration which gave a daily dose of 1000 mg/kg (twice that of the high dose in the first study). Thus, although the amount of drug dosed was high, absorption occurred over a period of hours and a peak urine concentration was avoided. At the end of the 13 weeks the animals were killed and the bladders examined. There was no epithelial hyperplasia.

*(ii) Dogs* In the 13 week study in dogs there were no clinical signs related to practolol treatment. Blood samples, for haematology and biochemistry, and urine samples were taken at regular intervals and no significant differences from controls were observed. The eyes of all animals were examined by direct ophthalmoscopy at intervals and no treatment-related effects were seen. All animals received a full necropsy, major organs were weighed and all major systems, including eyes, were taken for histological examination. There were no changes which could be attributed to practolol.

In the 52 week study, three dogs/sex/group were killed after 26 weeks and four/sex/group after 52 weeks. No clinical effects related to practolol were observed. Body weight gains in the middle dose group females (50 mg/kg) were reduced in the final 40 weeks of treatment. Regular blood samples, for haematology and clinical chemistry, and urine samples were taken throughout the study and the eyes were examined. No treatment-related effects were observed. Arterial blood pressure, heart rate and electrocardiograms were recorded in the control and highest dose groups prior to treatment and at one, three and six months treatment. Heart rates in the practolol-treated animals were 34% lower than controls. This was an expected pharmacological effect of the compound. Blood pressure and electrocardiograms showed no treatment-related effects. At the end of the 26 and 52 weeks dosing periods all animals were killed, the major organs were weighed and major systems sampled for histological examination. There were no changes which could be related to practolol treatment.

A 4 week intravenous toxicity study in dogs at doses of 10 mg/kg/day practolol did not produce any treatment-related effects.

*(c) Teratogenic studies*

Half of the rats and rabbits in each study were killed on the day prior to normal parturition, the foetuses removed and stained with alizarin for examination of the skeleton. The remaining rats were allowed to litter and rear the offspring to weaning. No teratogenic effects were seen in either species.

*(d) Ocular Toxicity*

In the first study two rabbits received 2 drops of a 10% solution of practolol into one eye, the other served as a control. The eyes were observed at 10, 30 and 60 minutes and there was no reaction to practolol. In the second study six rabbits received two drops of a 10% solution of practolol into one eye three times daily for three weeks and two drops of the vehicle into the contralateral eye for the same period. The eyes were examined daily and no changes relating to practolol were observed.

*(e) Oncogenicity Studies*

In the 18 month study in mice the animals were dosed by catheter for the first four months; thereafter the drug was incorporated into the diet for 14 months. Body weight gains and mortality rates were similar in control and dosed animals, and deaths during the study were from spontaneous diseases known to occur in the strain. Four dosed mice were not necropsied due to cannibalism. At the end of the study all animals were necropsied and examined histologically. The incidence of tumours in this study is shown in Table 8. There was no evidence of a carcinogenic effect or of any other histological change related to treatment with practolol. In the 104 week

TABLE 8. Incidence of tumours in 80 week oncogenicity study with practolol in mice

| Organ | Males Control N = 25 | 20 mg/kg 23 | 100 mg/kg 24 | Females Control 24 | 20 mg/kg 24 | 100 mg/kg 25 |
|---|---|---|---|---|---|---|
| Bone Marrow | 2 | 0 | 0 | 0 | 0 | 0 |
| Bone | 0 | 1 | 0 | 0 | 0 | 0 |
| Harderian gland | 1 | 1 | 1 | 0 | 0 | 0 |
| Liver | 4 | 1 | 3 | 0 | 1 | 0 |
| Lung | 2 | 2 | 4 | 2 | 5 | 3 |
| Lymph node | 0 | 4 | 1 | 4 | 3 | 5 |
| Skin | 1 | 0 | 0 | 0 | 0 | 0 |
| Spleen | 2 | 0 | 0 | 1 | 1 | 2 |
| Testes | 1 | 3 | 0 | — | — | — |
| Thymus | 0 | 0 | 1 | 0 | 3 | 2 |
| Thyroid | 0 | 1 | 0 | 0 | 0 | 0 |
| Uterus | — | — | — | 1 | 1 | 1 |
| Total | 13 | 13 | 10 | 8 | 14 | 13 |

TABLE 9. Incidence of tumours in 104 week oncogenicity study with practolol in rats

| | Males | | | Females | | |
|---|---|---|---|---|---|---|
| Organ | Control N = 20 | 0.04% 20 | 0.2% 20 | Control 20 | 0.04% 20 | 0.2% 19 |
| Adipose tissue | 0 | 1 | 1 | 0 | 0 | 0 |
| Adrenal | 0 | 2 | 2 | 1 | 0 | 0 |
| Bone | 0 | 0 | 1 | 0 | 0 | 0 |
| Bone Marrow | 1 | 0 | 1 | 0 | 3 | 1 |
| Intestine | 0 | 0 | 0 | 0 | 0 | 1 |
| Liver | 0 | 0 | 0 | 0 | 0 | 0 |
| Lung | 3 | 0 | 0 | 0 | 0 | 0 |
| Lymph node | 0 | 1 | 4 | 0 | 3 | 0 |
| Mammary gland | 0 | 1 | 1 | 8 | 8 | 8 |
| Ovary | — | — | — | 1 | 0 | 1 |
| Pancreas | 1 | 0 | 1 | 0 | 0 | 0 |
| Parathyroid | 0 | 0 | 0 | 0 | 0 | 1 |
| Pituitary | 1 | 8 | 1 | 11 | 10 | 12 |
| Skin | 4 | 1 | 3 | 1 | 0 | 0 |
| Testes | 0 | 1 | 5 | — | — | — |
| Thymus | 3 | 1 | 2 | 3 | 1 | 1 |
| Thyroid | 2 | 0 | 1 | 0 | 0 | 2 |
| Uterus | — | — | — | 1 | 2 | 0 |
| Unknown origin | 0 | 0 | 0 | 0 | 2 | 0 |
| Total | 15 | 16 | 23 | 26 | 29 | 27 |

study in rats (Table 9) practolol was administered in the diet throughout the study. No clinical signs related to the drug were seen; body weight gains and mortality rates were similar in all groups. One dosed animal was not necropsied due to cannibalism. All other animals were given a full necropsy and histological examination. The incidence of tumours is shown in Table 9. There was no evidence of a carcinogenic effect or any other histological change related to practolol treatment.

*(f) Pharmacokinetics and Metabolism*

Blood samples taken from animals in chronic toxicity tests demonstrated that there was no sex difference in serum levels. Peak levels were achieved 3 h after dosing. There was linear relationship between dose and serum level and the half-life was 2.5–3.5 h (rats) and 3–4 h (dogs). On the basis of these studies it was concluded that a serum level of 2 $\mu$g/ml practolol would be sufficient to produce pharmacological activity. $^{14}$C practolol dosed to rats, mice and dogs showed that about 85% of the drug was absorbed after oral dosing and at doses of 10 or 20 mg/kg no more than 5% of the drug was metabolized. Excretion curves indicated that the higher the dose the less the

% recovery of $^{14}$C in the urine, suggesting a more pronounced metabolism of the $^{14}$C acetyl side chain at high levels. Studies in volunteers at I.C.I. indicated that there were no significant differences in pharmacokinetics and metabolism in animals and man. In man there was a linear relationship between dose and blood level; peak levels were achieved at about 7 h and the half-life was an average of 12 h. Ninety percent of practolol was excreted in the urine as unchanged drug and the remaining 10% was excreted as at least seven metabolites, two of which correlated with the two major metabolites in animals—hydroxy practolol and its glucuronide conjugate.

## 2. Additional Studies

After the withdrawal of practolol, due to adverse effects, many additional studies were carried out in different species in an attempt to establish an animal model of the unique adverse effects seen in man. Among the more important studies were the following.

### (a) Metabolic Studies

Practolol metabolism was studied in a variety of small animal species (Reeves *et al.*, 1979) and in human subjects who had shown side effects with practolol (Reeves *et al.*, 1978). No evidence was found of a link between abnormal metabolism and the practolol syndrome.

### (b) Nine Month Study in Marmosets (Callithrix jacchus)

This species was selected for study because it is a primate (no previous work had been done in a primate species), and unlike all other species (including man) it extensively deacetylated practolol (Reeves *et al.*, 1979). If the deacetylated metabolite was in some way a trigger for the development of the practolol syndrome, then a species producing it in large amounts might develop the symptoms. The study was also used to examine the metabolism and pharmacokinetics of practolol, gut function (by radiography), anti-nuclear factors and lymphocyte transformation, as well as *in vitro* studies with isolated ileum to examine responses to standard agonists. In addition, standard toxicological observations, including cardiac function, ophthalmology, clinical chemistry (including measurements of amino acids), haematology and histological examination were performed. No scientific clues were obtained that might help.

### (c) Additional Long Term Studies in the Rodent

These included a 21 month study in C57B1/10 mice and a 24 month study in Alpk-AP rats using groups of 65/sex/dose and dose levels of 0, 150 and

300 mg/kg/day practolol. No changes relating to the syndrome were detected.

*(d) Investigation of Tyrosine/Practolol Interaction*

The rare inherited metabolic disorder of tyrosine metabolism in man (Richner-Hanhart syndrome or tyrosinemia type II) is characterized by eye and skin lesions which bear some clinical resemblance to the adverse effects seen in man with practolol. The possibility of an effect of practolol in tyrosine metabolism was studied by feeding rats various regimens of diets with low protein, high tyrosine levels and dosing with practolol. These studies did not produce any change which resembled the adverse effects seen in man.

*(e) Studies on Immunological Function in Animals*

*Effects on T suppressor cells.* Mice (Balb/C and C57) were dosed with practolol 300–500 mg/kg for 12–18 months. The incidence of anti-nuclear antibody was similar in treated and controls, suggesting that in this species practolol did not induce a defect in T suppressor cells. The development of antibodies to polyvinylpyrrolidone (PVP) is enhanced if T suppressor cells are depressed or removed. Three strains of mice (DBA/2, CBA and Balb/C) were treated with practolol for up to 1 year, but no strain showed an enhanced antibody response to PVP.

The possible effect of practolol on T-effector cells was examined in marmosets (lymphocyte transformation to PHA), mice (oxazolone contact sensitivity) and rats (adjuvant arthritis). Practolol did not alter the response in any of the T-effector cell-dependent animal models. Finally, chronic peritonitis was induced in mice by injection of Freund's adjuvant and the effect of practolol pre-treatment evaluated. Practolol did not worsen the experimental peritonitis.

There is, therefore, no clear evidence from experimental studies that practolol modifies the immune system in a manner relevant to the practolol syndrome.

# IV. Clinical experience

## A. Pronethalol

### 1. Predictions Prior to Clinical Study

Pharmacological studies with pronethalol in animals were primarily concerned with its effects on the cardiovascular system. Pronethalol reduced heart rate and cardiac contractile force, and caused a varying reduction in blood pressure in proportion to the speed of parenteral injection. Pharmocological studies were also carried out to examine its effects on baroceptor reflexes, intestinal motility, respiratory rate and the central nervous system. From such pharmacological studies it was predicted:

(a) That pronethalol would reduce heart rate at rest, on exercise and during emotional stress, as well as cause a small fall in blood pressure.
(b) That it might in higher doses cause some disturbance of the central nervous system.

## 2. Early Clinical Studies

Pronethalol, which was formulated either as a parenteral solution of 50 mg in 5 ml or as a 100 mg tablet, was evaluated for its anti-arrhythmic actions, especially during anaesthesia and in the peri-operative management of phaeochromocytoma. Its effects were also studied on exercise tolerance in subjects with angina pectoris. It was shown to have a beneficial effect in both arrhythmias (Stock and Dale, 1963) and angina pectoris (Dornhorst and Robinson, 1962; Alleyne et al., 1964).

## 3. Prediction and Experience

The negative chronotropic actions, as well as the beneficial effects in arrhythmias and angina pectoris, were predicted prior to study in man. A major unexpected effect of pronethalol was the occasional reduction in cardiac function leading to left ventricular failure. Cardiac failure was not predicted from animal studies, but, with hindsight, could have been (Black, 1967). Pronethalol caused light-headedness, slight incoordination and sometimes nausea and vomiting in about 25% of patients. Paraesthesia and visual disturbances were observed at higher doses. These effects were not anticipated at therapeutic doses in man, but were not unexpected because pronethalol in doses of 200–300 mg/kg orally caused muscle twitching and convulsions in cats, dogs and monkeys. These effects were attributed to a non-specific toxic action. Finally, skin rashes were observed in six of 400 patients receiving pronethalol and these were not predicted from the animal studies.

Interestingly, no cases of bronchospasm were reported during the studies with pronethalol. The Clinical Trials Brochure cautions against its use in patients liable to bronchospasm, though there are no reported observations on effects on bronchial beta adrenoceptors in preclinical studies. The clinically significant anti-hypertensive effect of pronethalol was not predicted from animal studies.

### 4. Pronethalol and Oncogenicity

The oncogenic studies of pronethalol in mice have been described in detail. This led to its withdrawal and the likelihood of such an effect being observed in man will never be known.

# B. Propranolol

Propranolol was discovered in 1962 and was shown to be 10–20 times more potent than pronethalol. It had the same central nervous system effects as pronethalol but a much wider therapeutic margin because of its increased beta antagonist potency. It was shown to be an effective anti-arrhythmic, anti-anginal and anti-hypertensive agent. It is not oncogenic and no oncogenic effects have been observed in man after 20 years exposure.

### 1. Prediction Prior to Clinical Study

The main expectations concerning propranolol were that it would be better tolerated than pronethalol in regard to non-specific central nervous system effects which had been encountered in about 25% of pronethalol-treated subjects. The absence of an oncogenic effect in susceptible mice indicated a greater safety margin for human subjects receiving propranolol over a prolonged period. It was anticipated that it would have a similar anti-arrhythmic and anti-anginal effect to pronethalol, but, because of its enhanced specificity, would be better tolerated.

### 2. Early Clinical Studies

The initial recommended dose of propranolol was 30 mg three times daily, or 1–4 mg intravenously. In the first 40 cases studied there was one case of heart failure, one case of erythematous rash and two reports of insomnia.

The widespread use of propranolol subsequently has been associated with a wide variety of unwanted effects, mostly those due to its pharmacological action. These are bradycardia, hypotension, cold extremities and broncho-spasm in susceptible subjects. The incidence of heart failure in patients with angina reported in all publications between 1965 and 1969 was 28 from a population of 2,137 cases studied, i.e. 1.3% incidence.

Central nervous system effects are common and comprise muzziness, dizziness, nausea, vomiting, mental confusion, insomnia and vivid dreams. Fatigue and lethargy are also common. Skin rashes and bowel disturbances are occasionally encountered.

3. Prediction and Experience

*(a) Efficacy*

The predicted beneficial effect of propranolol in controlling arrhythmias and angina pectoris were amply confirmed. The most striking beneficial effect in prolonging life in survivors after acute myocardial infarction, though predicted in 1960 by Black, was not proven until 1982 ($\beta$-Blocker Heart Attack Study Group, 1981; Lewis, 1982). The beneficial therapeutic effect of propranolol in essential hypertension, thyrotoxicosis, migraine, hypertrophic obstructive cardiomyopathy and glaucoma, as well as in selected forms of anxiety state, were not predicted prior to clinical study. Though $\beta$-antagonists are now used as primary therapy for treatment in essential hypertension, it was at least seven years after Prichard's initial observations (Prichard and Gillam, 1964) before this became generally accepted.

*(b) Unwanted Effects*

The possibility of marked adverse haemodynamic effects in susceptible patients was not foreseen prior to clinical study. In the very early studies clinically significant acute reductions in blood pressure were observed following intravenous injection of propranolol (1–5 mg). Subsequently, extreme caution was urged when using propranolol intravenously, especially for the management of arrhythmias in the peri-infarction period (Stephen, 1966). No indication was given that the administration of propranolol might prolong atrioventricular conduction time, particularly in patients with class 1 or class 2 heart block. Furthermore, no reference was made in the early publications on both pronethalol and propranolol concerning possible adverse effects on respiratory function in susceptible patients. The first published reference to this possibility was in 1964 (McNeil, 1964). The need for caution in using propranolol in patients with hypoglycaemia or metabolic acidosis was not considered prior to clinical study.

As a consequence of the early clinical experiences with propranolol, the subsequent laboratory testing of $\beta$-antagonists has become much more extensive and sophisticated. This is especially the case in regard to assessing their ancillary pharmacological properties and their haemodynamic profile as well as their effects on respiratory smooth muscle. It is doubtful if these additional studies improved the prediction of effects in man.

## C. Practolol

The discovery and development of practolol was based on an attempt to reduce the non-specific central nervous system effects observed with both pronethalol and propranolol. These central nervous system effects were thought to be related to the high lipid solubility of these compounds, possibly resulting in high concentrations within the central nervous system. At about the same time, Vaughan Williams (1966) published his observations that both these drugs were potent local anaesthetics and he speculated that this non-beta blocking property might contribute to both the anti-arrhythmic and cardiac depressant actions of pronethalol and propranolol. He showed that propranolol depressed the rate of rise and overshoot of the transmembrane action potential and coined the term "quinidine-like activity". As a result of these speculations and observations, a programme of chemical synthesis was initiated, specifically aimed at producing a $\beta$-antagonist with low lipid solubility. It was known at that time that the ethanolamine $\beta$-antagonist, sotalol, was very water soluble, so oxypropranolamine analogues were made in an attempt to discover potent $\beta$-antagonists of low lipophilicity. Practolol was one of the earliest synthesized and shown not to have local anaesthetic activity or direct cardio-depressant properties. The decision was made to compare the effects of practolol in man with those of propranolol and its dextro-isomer in order to establish the clinical relevance of the quinidine-like activity or membrane stabilizing properties of $\beta$-antagonists (Barrett, 1973). During the pharmacological evaluation of practolol in animals, it was discovered that it blocked the cardiac actions of isoprenaline at doses which had no effect on the vasodepressor actions of isoprenaline (Dunlop and Shanks, 1968).

This observation generated great excitement since it was the first indication that it might be possible selectively to antagonize cardiac adrenoceptors without antagonizing bronchial adrenoceptors. These observations were made prior to the hypothesis developed by Lands *et al.* (1967) concerning the existence of $\beta_1$ and $\beta_2$ receptors.

### 1. Predictions Prior to Clinical Study

It was anticipated that practolol would be an effective antagonist at cardiac adrenoceptors but not cause bronchospasm in susceptible subjects. It was also predicted that it would be an effective anti-anginal and anti-arrhythmic agent with an increased margin of safety. The marked difference in haemodynamic profile was not predicted.

### 2. Clinical Experience

Practolol was introduced into clinical study in 1967 and was soon shown to possess both anti-anginal and anti-arrhythmic effects. Furthermore, it was shown to be much better tolerated than propranolol in patients liable to bronchospasm (McNeil, 1971). There was a general impression amongst

TABLE 10. General unwanted effects in 2100 patients treated with practolol

| Effect | No. of Patients | Treatment stopped |
|---|---|---|
| Constipation | 44 | — |
| Diarrhoea | 4 | 3 |
| Increased appetite | 2 | — |
| Gastric upset | 4 | 1 |
| Nausea | 10 | 5 |
| Vomiting | 11 | 4 |
| Abdominal distension | 1 | 1 |
| Headaches | 4 | 1 |
| Dizziness, unsteadiness | 7 | 1 |
| Fatigue, lethargy, malaise | 6 | 2 |
| Depression | 2 | 1 |
| Vivid dreams | 2 | — |
| Rash | 7 | 5 |
| Paraesthesiae | 3 | 1 |
| Miscellaneous | 3 | 1 |

clinicians studying the drug, that it was better tolerated than propranolol especially in regard to central nervous system effects (see Table 10). The haemodynamic effects of practolol were markedly different from propranolol, particularly when given intravenously to patients in the peri-infarction period, or in heart failure (Jewitt and Croxson, 1971; Gibson et al., 1968).

There is no doubt that this impression of a more acceptable haemodynamic profile with lesser effects on respiratory function without evidence of diminished clinical efficacy all combined to give the impression that practolol had a better risk–benefit ratio than either propranolol or oxprenolol, the only other beta antagonists available at that time (Drug and Therapeutics Bulletin, 1971). The unwanted effects of practolol were summarized by Wiseman (1971). Of 223 patients receiving practolol (100–400 mg daily) for 6–24 months, the commonest side effects were constipation (14) and nausea (4). Skin rashes were not commented upon in this subgroup, though in the total number of patients studied (2,100) rashes were reported in only seven. Clearly, when practolol was introduced into the market in June, 1970, it appeared to be at least as effective as propranolol and better tolerated. The only side effects listed in the early practolol literature are constipation, nausea, vomiting and occasional skin rashes.

## 3. Unwanted Effects Detected Post-marketing

During the first two years of widespread use, the only change in the incidence of side effects associated with practolol usage was an increase in reports of skin rashes and sparse reports of skin rashes associated with fever and joint pains. In such patients, it was advised that the drug should be discontinued. Raftery and Denman (1973) observed that three anginal patients treated with practolol developed arthralgia, rash, fever associated with elevated ESR and positive tests for LE cells and anti-nuclear antibody. These symptoms developed after 4–6 months treatment with 600–1200 mg practolol daily. In a follow-up study, Pugh *et al.* (1976) reported an incidence of 11% of anti-nuclear factor (ANF) in 71 patients receiving practolol for an average period of six months.

A more recent controlled study (Jachuck *et al.*, 1977) compared the incidence of various auto-antibodies in 51 patients receiving practolol for ischaemic heart disease and dysrhythmias, with 204 similar patients not receiving practolol. ANF was detected in 24% of female and 16% of male patients receiving practolol, but only 5% of female and 4% of male patients who were not receiving practolol. During this time the practolol multicentre post-infarction trial was in progress involving 1500 patients receiving the drug. Tests for ANF in this large group showed an incidence of about 10% but it was obvious that the clinical manifestations of the practolol-induced LE syndrome were very rare.

In 1974 a unique constellation of symptoms and signs associated with practolol administration was reported (Felix *et al.*, 1974; Wright, 1975). The chief features of what was to become known as the oculomucocutaneous syndrome were:

(1) Psoriasiform rash with hyperkeratosis of the palms and soles, with fissuring along the sides of the digits.
(2) An unusual form of keratoconjunctivitis sicca with characteristic and unique subconjunctival fibrotic changes associated with varying degrees of corneal ulceration leading to opacification and loss of vision in some cases.
(3) A bilateral secretory otitis media accompanied in a few patients with a sensori-neural type of deafness due to cochlear involvement.
(4) A unique type of sclerosing peritonitis in which the visceral peritoneum became thickened, enclosing the bowel in a matt of fibrous tissue.
(5) In a small number of cases there was also involvement of other serosal membranes resulting in fibrotic changes in the pleura and the pericardium.

## 4. Histopathology

Skin rash attributable to practolol is often described as psoriasiform, but exematous, lichenoid and mixed eruptions have also been described. Histologically, the practolol skin reaction comprises hyperkeratosis, with peculiar colloid bodies distributed through the epidermis to the horny layer. In the epidermis there is spongiosis, acanthosis, epidermotropism with

individual cell keratinization and liquefaction of the basal layer. A pleo-
morphic cellular infiltrate extending deep into the dermis with a mainly
perivascular distribution is observed.

Histological examination of the conjunctiva shows metablastic changes in
the surface epithelium associated with acanthosis and loss of goblet cells.
Chronic inflammatory changes resulting in sub-conjunctival fibrosis are also
observed.

Examination of material obtained from patients with sclerosing peritonitis
reveals a thick fibrous tissue comprising layers of coarse collagen bundles
interspersed with occasional fibroblasts and mononuclear cells. It must be
emphasized that this fibrosing peritonitis has nothing in common, clinically
or histologically, with retroperitoneal fibrosis.

## 5. Aetiology of Oculomucocutaneous Syndrome

Possible mechanisms considered are pharmacological, toxicological,
immunological or metabolic. The fact that this syndrome has not been
reported in patients receiving other $\beta$-antagonists makes it clear that the
syndrome associated with practolol administration is not due to beta blockade. Furthermore, over 200 patients with practolol-induced skin problems
have been transferred to other $\beta$-blockers and the skin condition has
resolved (Nicholls, 1976). If a conventional toxicological process were the
cause, then it should be possible to reproduce the syndrome in animals.
Prolonged administration of practolol in doses of up to 300 mg/kg/day for
18–24 months to rats, mice and hamsters did not reveal any serious toxicity
and certainly nothing resembling the human syndrome. Prolonged studies in
dogs and marmosets have also been unhelpful. In view of the low incidence
in man, detection of a similar incidence rate in animals would require huge
numbers.

The possibility that the syndrome has an immunological basis has been
widely discussed and has been postulated by some investigators. However,
the mechanism involved is still unknown.

## 6. Autoantibodies and the Oculomucocutaneous Syndrome

The association between practolol administration and the detection of
antinuclear factors has already been described. There is clearly a significant
increase in ANF in practolol-treated subjects.

Intercellular depositions of various immunoglobulins have also been
observed in tissue obtained from patients with skin and eye involvement.
Deposition of immunoglobulin (IgG) has been demonstrated in the intercellular region (Dahl *et al.*, 1975; Rahi *et al.*, 1976; Amos *et al.*, 1978). The only

finding to emerge from extensive studies on autoantibodies is that there is an increased incidence of antinuclear antibody in patients receiving practolol, but there is no clear evidence of an agreed association between the incidence of this antibody and tissue damage, nor is there evidence of such a relationship for other autoantibodies.

Lymphocyte function has been assessed in patients receiving practolol as well as those with the practolol syndrome. In the study by Behan *et al.* (1976) some depression of lymphocyte function was observed in 11 of 15 patients with practolol lesions, but in addition 5 of 6 patients who had been on practolol for two years without untoward effect, also had some depression. It should only be concluded therefore that there is an association between alteration of immune function and the administration of practolol, but not with practolol-induced side effects. Amos and Brigden (1976) observed that the phytohaemagglutinin (PHA) response of lymphocytes from 16 patients with severe eye damage was normal. Pugh *et al.* (1976) showed depressed lymphocyte responses in patients with the practolol syndrome, but only in those with a raised ESR and not necessarily with either practolol administration or the presence of anti-nuclear antibody. Interesting studies have also been reported on the results of challenge tests in an attempt to demonstrate an allergic reaction to practolol, and also on immune mechanisms directed against the drug (*vide supra*). In reviewing the papers in this area, Davies (1979) came to the conclusion that it is impossible to derive any meaningful conclusion from the various studies on immunological abnormalities associated with the practolol syndrome. Very few of the findings have received independent confirmation and difficulties of interpretation stem from the variables inherent in the problem.

The variables of particular importance are the nature of the side effect, the age and degree of medical instability of the patients, the period on and off the drug, as well as marked differences in techniques, or inadequate description of immunological techniques, including the absence of, or inadequate use of, controls. Perhaps, the clearest association is observed between the immunological phenomena and tissue damage produced by practolol administration. However, most of the immunological abnormalities reported are seen in patients who have taken practolol without untoward effect. Antibodies are produced to drugs and their metabolites in many situations, the classical one being that of penicillin. There is however no evidence that the presence of such circulating antibodies can be directly associated with drug-induced side effects, with the possible exception of the reagenic antibodies to penicillin. Clearly, autoantibodies will appear in response to marked tissue damage of several kinds and hence the relationship between the practolol syndrome and the various immunological abnormalities described remains unproven.

7. Practolol Metabolism

Metabolism of practolol has been studied extensively in man and several animal species. In man, rat, mouse and dog it is extensively and rapidly excreted unchanged in the urine. The minor metabolites in man are 3-hydroxypractolol and the de-acetylated analogue. The metabolic pattern in man is similar to rat and mouse which are the species most frequently used to study the toxicity of practolol. In studies of the metabolism of practolol by liver microsomal enzyme systems, it was shown that practolol binds covalently to macromolecules in the presence of oxygen and NADPH. The de-acetylated metabolite of practolol was a five times better substrate for causing covalent binding. It has been hypothesized that the covalent binding may result in an immunogenic complex arising from practolol metabolites, but despite clinical and experimental studies the aetiological mechanism for the practolol syndrome remains unknown.

# V. Conclusions

Beta antagonists, when first studied in man, represented a new type of specific pharmacological action. As with all novel specific agents, three questions arose:

(a) Would the pharmacological action seen in the laboratories be reproduced to the clinical benefit of patients?
(b) Based on animal studies, what hazards were likely to arise from the acute or prolonged effect of this type of pharmacological action (in this case prolonged beta blockade)?
(c) What hazards might this novel chemical structure induce, irrespective of its known pharmacological actions?

It must be emphasized that the majority of toxicological studies described here are only those carried out prior to use in man. Many other studies have been done since, but they are not relevant to a discussion on the predictive value of animal testing.

In the case of pronethalol, it was anticipated that it would reduce heart rate and possibly blood pressure when given acutely (Black, 1967). It was not anticipated that it would induce heart failure in certain patients. Pronethalol was known to cause impairment of central nervous system function in animals, so the reports of hallucinations, dizziness, dreams, etc. in the prolonged anti-anginal studies, whilst not accurately predicted, were not surprising. A major surprise was the association of thymic tumours in pronethalol-treated mice. As is emphasized in the text, pronethalol is not a predictable carcinogen in strains of mice other than the Alderley Park strain, and is not carcinogenic in other animal species. Since pronethalol was soon withdrawn from human use, the overall predictive value of the Alderley Park mouse strain for carcinogenic potential in man cannot be determined and it may be that pronethalol's oncogenic effect in that strain of mice is due to an indirect rather than a direct action (Newberne, 1977).

The unwanted pharmacological side effects, due to propranolol administration, of bronchospasm, cold extremities and fatigue, were not predicted but were not unexpected. Practolol was expected to have less effect on bronchial tone than propranolol and this was shown to be the case (McNeil, 1971). Its lesser effects on heart rate were also anticipated, but the very clear difference in haemodynamic profile was not anticipated. Propranolol when given intravenously in the peri-infarction period, caused marked reduction in heart rate and cardiac output, whereas practolol had much less effect. Practolol was regarded as much safer for acute administration in this situation (Jewitt and Croxson, 1971). Propranolol does cause a dose-dependent reduction in cardiac contractile force, which is due, in low doses, to blockade of endogenous sympathetic tone and in high doses to its membrane stabilizing properties (Fitzgerald et al., 1972). The lesser haemodynamic effect of practolol could be due either to PAA, absence of membrane stabilizing properties, or to its $\beta_1$ selectivity. Recent studies with atenolol, which has a similar haemodynamic profile to propranolol, show that when given intravenously within 6 h of an acute myocardial infarction, it is well tolerated and can reduce symptoms (Yusef et al., 1983). Previously, however, practolol was regarded as the best tolerated beta blocker because: (1) it caused much smaller haemodynamic changes and reduction in heart rate than propranolol; (2) it had few central nervous system side effects; and (3) it caused less fatigue. None of these differences were explicitly recognized prior to human study. The explicit expectation was a lesser effect on bronchial tone in asthmatic subjects, and this prediction was fulfilled.

By far the greatest failure of extensive animal testing for prediction of serious side effects is seen in the case of practolol. From the detailed descriptions of the animal studies carried out both before and after the practolol syndrome was described, it is clear that animal studies have not been helpful either in predicting or explaining the oculomucocutaneous syndrome. The practolol syndrome was a rare occurrence in man and its rarity may contribute to the problem of inducing it in other species.

## References*

Ahlquist, R. P. (1948). A study of the adrenotropic receptors. *Am. J. Physiol.* **153**, 586–600.

*"Alderlin", "Eraldin" and "Inderal" are trade marks, the property of Imperial Chemical Industries PLC.

Alcock, S. J. and Bond, P. A. (1964). Observations on the toxicity of "Alderlin" (pronethalol) in laboratory animals. *Proc. Europ. Soc. Study Drug Tox.* **IV**, 30–37.

Alleyne, G. A. O., Dickinson, C. J., Dornhorst, A. C., Fulton, R. M., Green, K. G., Hill, I. D., Hurst, P., Laurence, D. R., Pilkington, T., Prichard, B. N. C., Robinson, B. and Rosenheim, M. L. (1963). The effect of pronethalol in angina pectoris. *Br. Med. J.* (**ii**), 1226–1229.

Amos, H. E. and Brigden, W. D. (1976). Immunological changes and practolol. *Lancet,* **II**, 1298.

Amos, H. E., Lake, B. G. and Artis, J. (1978). Possible role of antibody specific for a practolol metabolite in the pathogenesis of oculomucocutaneous syndrome. *Br. Med. J.* **I**, 402.

Assem, E. S. K. and Banks, R. A. (1973). Practolol induced drug eruption. *Proc. Roy. Soc. Med.* **66**, 179.

Barrett, A. M. and Fitzgerald, J. D. (1968). What is a $\beta$-blocker. *Am. J. Cardiol.* **76**, 712–714.

Barrett, A. M. (1973). The pharmacology of beta-adrenoceptor antagonists. *In* "Recent Advances in Cardiology", (J. Hamer, Ed). 6th ed. pp. 289–328. Churchill Livingstone, Edinburgh and London.

Behan, P. O., Behan, W. M. H., Zacharias, F. J. and Nicholls, J. T. (1976). Immunological abnormalities in patients who had the oculomucocutaneous syndrome associated with practolol therapy. *Lancet,* **II**, 984.

Beta-blocker Heart Attack Study Group (1981) The beta-blocker heart attack trial. *J.A.M.A.* **246**, 2073–2074.

Black, J. W. (1967) The predictive value of animal tests in relation to drugs affecting the cardiovascular system in man. *In* Wolstenholme, G. and Porter, R. Eds. Drug responses in man, pp. 111–124. J. and A. Churchill, Ltd., London.

Black, J. W. and Stephenson, J. S. (1962) Pharmacology of a new adrenergic beta blocking compound (nethalide). *Lancet,* **2**, 311–313.

Black, J. W., Duncan, W. A. M. and Shanks, R. G. (1965) Comparison of some properties of pronethalol and propranolol. *Br. J. Pharmacol.,* **25**, 577–591.

Brown, P., Baddeley, H., Read, A. E., Davies, J. D. and McGarry, J. (1974) Sclerosing peritonitis, an unusual reaction to a beta-adrenergic blocking drug (practolol). *Br. Med. J.,* **I**, 598.

Cruickshank, J. (1981) The clinical importance of cardioselectivity and lipophilicity in beta blockers. *Am. Heart J,* **100**, 160–178.

Dahl, M. G. C., Felix, R. H., Ive, F. A. and Wilkinson, D. S. (1975) Immunologic aspects of practolol-induced lupus erythematosus. *J. Invest. Dermatol.,* **64**, 299.

Dale, H. H. (1966) On some physiological actions of ergot *J. Physiol. (Lond.),* **34**, 163–206.

Davies, G. E. (1979) Adverse reactions to practolol. "Drugs and Immune Responsiveness", Eds. Turk and Parker, 1979, p. 199.

Dornhurst, A. C. and Robinson, B. F. (1962) Clinical pharmacology of a beta-blocking agent (nethalide) *Lancet,* **2**, 314–316.

*Drug and Therapeutics Bulletin* (1971) Oxprenol and practolol: new beta blockers, **9**, 1–3.

Dunlop, D. and Shanks, R. G. (1968) Selective blockade of adrenoceptive beta-receptors in the heart. *Br. J. Pharmacol.,* **32**, 201–218.

Felix, R. H., Ive, F. A. and Dahl, M. G. C. (1974) Cutaneous and ocular reactions to practolol. *Br. Med. J.,* **4**, 321–324.

Fitzgerald, J. D. (1969) Perspectives in adrenergic beta-receptor blockade. *Clin. Pharmacol. Ther.,* **10**, 292–306.

Fitzgerald, J. D. (1982) The effect of different classes of beta antagonists on clinical and experimental hypertension. *Clin. Exp. Hyper.* Theory and Practice, **A4** (1–2), 101–123.

Fitzgerald, J. D., Wale, J. L. and Austin, M. (1972) The haemodynamic effects of (±)-propranolol, dexpropranolol, oxprenolol, practolol and sotalol in anaesthetised dogs. *Eur. J. Pharm.*, **17**, 123–134.

Gibson, D. G., Balcon, R. and Sowton, E. (1968) Clinical use of ICI 50,172 as anti-dysrhythmic agent in heart failure. *Br. Med. J.*, **3**, 161–163.

Green, K. G. (1975) Improvement in prognosis of myocardial infarction by long term beta-adrenoceptor blockade using practolol. *Br. Med. J.*, **3**, 735–740.

Jachuck, S. J., Stephenson, J., Bird, T., Jackson, F. S. and Clark, F. (1977) Practolol-induced autoantibodies and their relation to oculocutaneous complications. *Postgrad. Med. J.*, **53**, 75.

Jewitt, D. and Croxson, R. (1971) Practolol in the management of cardiac dysrhythmias following myocardial infarction and cardiac surgery. *Postgrad. Med.*, **5**, **47** (suppl.), 25–29.

Lands, A. M., Arnold, A., McAuliff, J. P. et al (1967) Differentiation of receptor systems activated by sympathomimetic amines. *Nature*, **214**, 597–598.

Lewis, J. A. (1982) β-Blockade after myocardial infarction—a statistical view. *Br. J. clin. Pharmacol.*, **14**, 15S–21S.

Lish, P. M., Weikel, J. H. and Dungan, K. W. (1965) Pharmacological and toxicological properties of two new beta-adrenergic receptor antagonists. *J. Pharmacol. Exp. Ther.*, **149**, 161–173.

McNeil, R. S. (1964) Effect of a beta adrenergic blocking agent on asthmatics. *Lancet*, **2**, 1101–1103.

McNeil, R. S. (1971) The effects of beta antagonists on the bronchi. *Postgrad. Med. J.* **47** (suppl.), 14–16.

Moran, N. C. and Perkins, M. E. (1958) Adrenergic blockade of the mammalian heart by a dichloro analog of isoproterenol *J. Pharmacol.*, **124**, 223–237.

Newberne, J. W., Newberne, P. M., Gibson, J. P., Huffman, K. K. and Palolpoli, F. P. (1977) Lack of carcinogenicity of oxprenolol, a β-adrenergic blocking agent. *Toxicol. Appl. Pharmacol.*, **41**, 535–542.

Nicholls, J. T. (1976) Adverse effects of practolol. *Ann. Clin. Res.*, **8**, 229.

Orton, T. C. and Lowery, C. (1977) Irreversible protein binding of [$^{14}$C]-practolol metabolites to hamster liver microsomes. *Br. J. Pharmac.*, **60**, 319P.

Paget, G. E. (1963) Carcinogenic action of pronethalol. *Br. Med. J.*, **2**, 1266.

Powell, C. E. and Slater, J. H. (1958) Blocking of inhibitory adrenergic receptors by a dichloroanalog of isoproterenol. *J. Pharmacol.*, **122**, 480–488.

Prichard, B. N. C. and Gillam, P. M. S. (1964) The treatment of hypertension with propranolol. *Br. Med. J.*, **2**, 725–727.

Pugh, S., Pelton, B., Raftery, E. B. and Denman, A. M. (1976) Abnormal lymphocyte function is secondary to drug-induced autoimmunity. *Ann. Rheum. Dis.*, **35**, 344.

Raftery, E. B. and Denman, A. M. (1973) Systemic lupus erythematous syndrome induced by practolol. *Br. Med. J.*, **2**, 452.

Rahi, A. H . S., Chapman, C. M., Garner, A. and Wright, P. (1976) Pathology of practolol-induced ocular toxicity. *Br. J. Ophthal.*, **60**, 312

Reeves, P. R., Case, D. E., Jepson, H. T., McCormick, D. J., Nicholls, J. T., Felix, R. H., Holt, P. J. L., Zacharias, F. J. and Fluke, R. W. (1978) Practolol metabolism 11. Metabolism in human subjects. *J. Pharmacol. Exp. Ther.*, **205**, 489–498.

Reeves, P. R., McCormick, D. J. and Jepson, H. T. (1979) Practolol metabolism in various small animal species. *Xen. biotica*, **9**, 453–458.

Riddell, D. H., Schull, L. G., Frist, T. F. and Baker, T. D. (1963) Experiences with pheochromocytoma in 21 patients. Use of dichloro-iso-proterenol hydrochloride for cardiac arrhythmias. *Ann. Surg.*, **157**, 980–988.

Stephen, S. (1966) Unwanted effects of propranolol. *Am. J. Cardiol.*, **18**, 463–467.

Stock, J. P. P. and Dale, N. (1963) Beta-adrenergic receptor blockade in cardiac arrhythmias. *Br. Med. J.*, **2**, 1230–1233.

Tucker, M. J. (1968) Observations relating to the carcinogenic action of pronethalol ("Alderlin") *Proc. Europ. Soc. Study Drug Tox.*, **X**, 175–182.

Vaughan Williams, E. M. (1966) Mode of action of $\beta$-receptor antagonists on cardiac muscle. *Am. J. Cardiol.*, **18**, 399–405.

Wiseman, R. A. (1971) Practolol—accumulated data on unwanted effects. *Postgrad. Med. J.*, **47** (suppl.), 68–71.

Wright, P. (1975) Untoward effect associated with practolol administration. Oculomucocutaneous syndrome. *Br. Med. J.*, **1**, 595–598.

Yusef, S., Ramsdale, D., Rossi, P., Peto, R., Pearson, M., Sterry, H., Turse, L., Moturani, R., Parish, S., Gray, R., Bennett, D., Bray, C. and Slight, P. (1983) Early intravenous atenolol treatment in suspected acute myocardial infarction. *New Engl. J. Md.* (in press).

## Addendum

## The Practolol Scheme

Some aspects of the oculomucocutaneous syndrome attributable to practolol began to come to light in June, 1974. Practolol was restricted to use in hospitals only for certain specific short-term indications from September, 1975. ICI sought independent legal opinion as to its legal liability. The clear opinion of two Queen's Counsel was that ICI had no legal liability in respect of reactions suffered by patients treated with practolol.

Despite the absence of legal liability, ICI decided to set up a scheme to assist those patients who suffered permanent injury as a result of taking practolol. The practolol scheme was devised with the objective of ensuring speedy consideration of cases (particularly as many of the patients were elderly and seriously ill because of their heart condition). In addition, it was intended to provide reasonable levels of payment and equality of treatment, even though it was not initially known how many cases attributable to practolol might arise. The levels of payment were related to the amounts which a court could be expected to award if legal liability were to be established. The main factors influencing the final settlement were, the degree of permanent damage and the patient's age. Payments have also been adjusted to take account of individual expenses and for inflation. Patients were advised to consult their doctors and then to contact ICI, preferably through a solicitor of their choice. ICI agreed to pay all reasonable legal and medical costs incurred in investigating a claim and obtaining reports from medical specialists.

# 6

# Tamoxifen

MARY J. TUCKER, H. K. ADAM, J. S. PATTERSON

*ICI PLC, Pharmaceuticals Division, Alderley Park,
Macclesfield, Cheshire, England*

## I. Summary

Tamoxifen ("Nolvadex") is the trans (Z)-isomer of a triphenylethylene (Z) - 2 - [4 - (1,2 - diphenyl - 1 - butenyl)phenoxy] - N - N - dimethylethanamine which was first used in breast cancer in women in the late 1960's. Preclinical studies began in 1964 and continued for more than ten years. The studies included detailed toxicological studies in rats, dogs and monkeys for periods up to six months and several longer term studies in mice for periods between 12 and 15 months.

In general there were no significant toxicological effects other than those found in the reproductive tract. Since tamoxifen behaved as an oestrogen in some species and an anti-oestrogen in others, many studies were done comparing the effects of tamoxifen with known oestrogens and anti-oestrogens to elucidate the mechanism of the effects. Biliary stasis was seen in dogs but only at doses which are very high for a compound with endocrine activity (75 mg/kg/day). Benign gonadal tumours and bone changes were seen in mice at high doses and these were shown to be related to *oestrogenic* activity. The drug showed no mutagenic activity when tested using an *in vitro* liver metabolizing system and using bacteria capable of detecting both base pair and frameshift mutations (Ames test); no dominant lethal effect was observed. In teratogenic studies all doses above 2 mg/kg produced an incidence of irregular ossification of ribs in foetal rats. This was related to the *anti-oestrogenic* effect in the dam preventing uterine development and since this effect disappeared in the early neo-natal period it was not considered to be a teratogenic effect. Tamoxifen has now been used in breast cancer for more than ten years and its clinical use continues to increase. It is one of a few novel therapies introduced into cancer therapy in the 1970's and its use is enhanced by the very low incidence of serious side effects. The preclinical experiments were protracted for an anti-cancer agent because tamoxifen was originally developed as an oral contraceptive agent and because of the variable pharmacology in different species; in general the absence of significant toxic effects has proven to be a good prediction for the effects in man.

## II. Introduction

The biochemical mechanisms underlying the action of oestrogens at the molecular level are not fully understood. Hence the pharmacology of tamoxifen can best be described in terms of its ability to act in a manner similar to oestrogens (oestrogenic) or to antagonize the action of oestrogen (anti-oestrogenic). Tamoxifen can behave as a pure agonist, a partial agonist or a pure antagonist, the response elicited depending on the species, dose or target organ being examined. The wide variety of actions, and the resultant effects of these, demands that each species be examined separately.

It is also worth pointing out that the pharmacology of the molecule is dictated by the stereochemistry about the central double bond. Tamoxifen (ICI 46,474), the pure trans-isomer, is the active ingredient of "Nolvadex". ICI 47,699 is the corresponding cis-isomer and has a distinct and different pharmacological profile from tamoxifen.

Non-steroidal anti-oestrogens of the triarylalkene group were of considerable interest during the 1960's as agents for terminating pregnancy by preventing implantation of the blastocyst in rats. One compound—clomiphene citrate (Clomid, Merrell)—was widely used in the treatment of infertility. Other compounds were introduced to clinical usage as potential successors to Clomid and these included ICI 46,474 which has the generic name tamoxifen (USAN tamoxifen citrate), proprietary name "Nolvadex". *

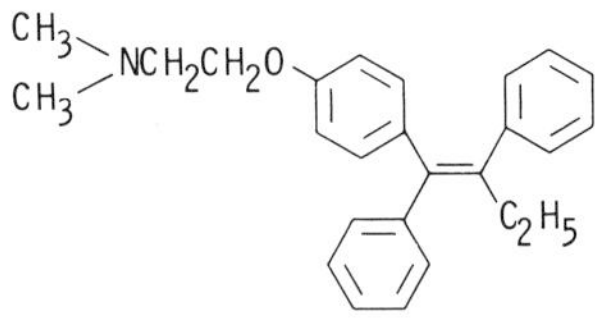

FIG. 1. Chemical structure of tamoxifen.

Tamoxifen (Fig. 1) is the trans (Z)-isomer of a triphenylethylene (Z)-2-[4-(1,2-diphenyl-1-butenyl)phenoxy]-N-N-dimethylethanamine; the corresponding cis (E)-isomer is a weakly oestrogenic compound, and less than 1% is present in "Nolvadex". The molecular weight of tamoxifen is 563.6 and the

* "Nolvadex" is a trade mark, the property of Imperial Chemical Industries-PLC.

molecular formula $C_{26}H_{29}NOC_6H_8O_7$. It is a white, odourless, crystalline powder which is only slightly soluble in water and is stable for more than five years when protected from light and moisture.

## III. Preclinical studies

### A. Rats

In the rat vagina tamoxifen has weak partial agonist activity at high doses. 41 mg/kg/day was the median $ED_{50}$ required to produce cornification in ovariectomized animals, whilst complete cornification could not be obtained. At lower doses the drug behaved as an antagonist in that it blocked the effect of a cornifying dose of oestradiol when the two substances were administered together. When dosed orally to immature female rats the effect on uterine weight demonstrated agonist activity when dosed alone, and antagonist activity when administered with oestradiol. These effects occurred over the same dose range (Fig. 2). The partial agonist effect was confirmed on subcutaneous dosing, where the maximal increase in uterine weight (induced by tamoxifen doses in the range 0.05 to 0.5 mg/kg/day × 3) was only two-thirds that produced by oestradiol (Jordan, 1976). Detailed studies on the uterus of rats whose uterine weight had been increased by tamoxifen or oestradiol showed that, as well as the quantitative difference in response, there were qualitative differences in mitotic counts and endometrial thickness (Clark *et al.*, 1978) or glycogen-like granules (Ljungkuist and Terenius, 1972).

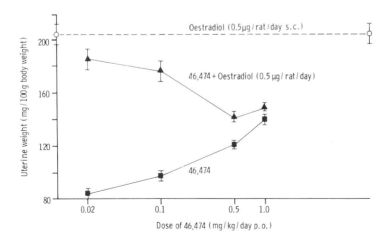

FIG. 2. Effect of ICI 46,474 on uterine weight of rats.

Tamoxifen terminates pregnancy in rats if dosed (0.03 mg/kg/day) over the first four days post mating. It is believed that this effect is due to antagonism of the oestradiol surge which is essential in the rat for implantation. In addition the inhibition of ovulation by tamoxifen is believed to be due to a feedback control mechanism at the hypothalamo-pituitary axis since it has been shown that tamoxifen can inhibit synthesis of oestradiol in the ovary (Watson et al., 1975). The oral $LD_{50}$ in rats is approximately 2000 mg/kg and the intravenous $LD_{50}$ is 62.5 mg/kg.

The first toxicity test with tamoxifen in this species was a three month oral administration test completed in 1963. Four groups, each of ten male and ten female rats of the Alderley Park strain 1 (Alpk/AP) were dosed daily by gavage at 0, 2, 20 and 100 mg/kg body weight tamoxifen for three months. The doses were selected on the basis that 2 mg/kg is 50–100 times the dose required to inhibit ovulation in the rat. Blood samples were taken for haematological examination from control and 100 mg/kg groups, predose and at six and 12 weeks. Urine samples were collected predose and at six weeks. At the end of treatment the animals were given a full post mortem examination, the major organs were weighed and samples of major tissues taken for histological examination.

Growth rate was depressed, to a similar degree, in all the treated groups; the only other clinical sign observed was loss of hair on the neck. No abnormalities were seen in blood and urine samples. The weights of ovaries, testes, seminal vesicles and ventral prostate were all reduced, to a similar degree, in all three treated groups. Histologically significant changes were seen only in the reproductive tract of the treated animals. In the ovaries, corpora lutea were less numerous and of less recent origin than in controls and follicular cysts were increased, particularly at the lowest dose (Fig. 3). The uteri were reduced in size and the endometrium showed absence of glands and the lining epithelium reduced to a single layer of columnar cells with small areas of flattening and occasional squamous metaplasia at the lowest dose (2 mg/kg). The endometrial stroma was condensed, giving a more fibrous appearance (Fig. 4). The testes showed cessation of sperm maturation and the accessory sex organs were atrophic. These changes in males were dose dependent and were minimal at 2 mg/kg. The changes in the reproductive system were interpreted as an *anti-oestrogenic* effect related to inhibition of the positive feedback action of oestrogens on the hypothalamic/pituitary axis.

To confirm this interpretation a second test was designed to compare the effects of tamoxifen in the rat with those of the anti-oestrogenic compound clomiphene. This was completed in 1964. Three groups, each of 15 female Alpk/AP rats were dosed by gavage daily with 0.5 or 2 mg/kg tamoxifen or 4 mg/kg clomiphene. The animals were dosed for three months, after which

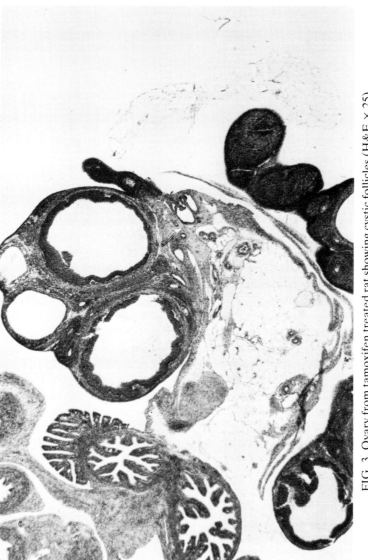

FIG. 3. Ovary from tamoxifen treated rat showing cystic follicles (H&E × 25).

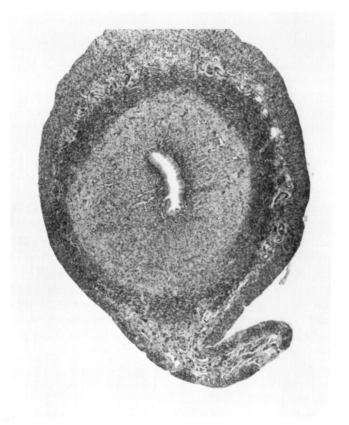

FIG 4. Uterus from tamoxifen treated rat showing condensed fibrous endometrial stroma (H&E × 25).

time five animals in each group were killed and necropsied. The drugs were withdrawn from the remaining ten animals in each group and they were left untreated for a further three months; at the end of this period the animals were killed and necropsied.

In the animals which were treated for three months, similar changes were seen in the reproductive tract of both clomiphene and tamoxifen treated animals. The ovaries showed reduced numbers of corpora lutea and increased numbers of follicular cysts; in the uterus endometrial glands were absent and the lining epithelium flattened. The changes were more marked in the animals treated with clomiphene. In the animals left untreated for three months the ovaries and uteri of tamoxifen treated rats had returned to normal but the changes were still present in the clomiphene treated animals although less marked than in the animals killed at three months.

These results were considered to confirm that the changes seen in the reproductive tract of tamoxifen treated rats were related to the *anti-oestrogenic* activity of the compound although clomiphene is also a partial oestrogen agonist. In 1977 a further study in rats was designed to support extended clinical use of tamoxifen and to establish a no-effect level for changes in the reproductive tract. Six groups, each of 25 male and 25 female Alpk/AP rats were dosed daily by stomach tube for six months at levels of 0, 0.5, 0.8, 2.4, 4.8 and 9.6 mg/kg body weight. Five animals of each sex in each group were killed and necropsied at three months, the remaining 20/sex/group at six months. Before treatment and at one, three and six months blood samples were taken for haematology and biochemistry, urine samples were collected, heart rate and blood pressure recorded and the eyes examined by ophthalmoscopy. Additional animals were dosed in parallel with the main study and used to examine coagulation factors. At the end of each period of treatment the designated animals were killed, the major organs weighed, and tissues taken for histological examination. Radiographs were taken of all animals killed at six months.

All treated groups showed a suppression of growth rate accompanied by a reduced food intake. There were no other clinical signs attributable to tamoxifen. No significant changes were seen in haematology, biochemistry or urine samples, or in the heart rate and blood pressure, and no abnormalities were found in the radiographs. Histological findings were confined to the reproductive tract and were similar to those seen in the first study; they were present at all dose levels but were minimal at the lowest dose (0.05 mg/kg).

Since the anti-oestrogenic compound clomiphene citrate has been shown to cause visual disturbances in man, but no morphological changes (Kistner, 1965; Roche *et al.*, 1967), and cataracts in adult rats (Clinical Pharmacology Therapeutics, 1967) and in foetal rats (Eneroth *et al.*, 1971) it was considered important to examine the effect of tamoxifen on the eye.

16 pregnant female Alpk/AP rats received a single subcutaneous dose of 200 mg/kg tamoxifen on Day 11 of pregnancy. 12 pregnant female Alpk/AP rats received a single subcutaneous dose of 50 mg/kg clomiphene citrate on Day 11 of pregnancy. 17 pregnant female Alpk/AP rats were used as controls and allowed to litter normally; the pups were killed Day 21 post partum.

Foetuses from the dams dosed with clomiphene and tamoxifen were delivered by Caesarian section on Day 22 of pregnancy and fostered onto untreated females which had recently littered. The pups were killed on Day 21 post partum. No cataracts were seen in the eyes of the control and tamoxifen groups; seven of 100 foetuses from dams dosed with clomiphene citrate had bilateral cataracts. It was considered that the effect of clomiphene on the eye is not related to its anti-oestrogenic activity but to the effect of the compound on cholesterol metabolism with accumulation of fatty material, probably desmosterol, in the lens. Tamoxifen slightly reduces cholesterol and desmosterol levels but does not alter liver cholesterol levels (Harper and Walpole, 1967).

## B. Dogs

The first toxicity test in this species was a three month oral administration test completed in 1964. Twenty eight beagles from the Alderley Park colony were used in four groups. The untreated control group included two males and two females; two groups of four males and four females received 1 or 10 mg/kg tamoxifen daily for three months and the highest dose groups of four males and four females received 50 mg/kg daily for two months then 75 mg/kg daily for one month. The doses were selected on the basis that 1 mg/kg is approximately ten times the level required to inhibit implantation in the dog. Blood samples for clinical chemistry were taken predose at 1, 10, 12 and 13 weeks. Urine samples were collected terminally. At the end of treatment all of the animals were killed and necropsied.

In the final month a male receiving 75 mg/kg died with severe jaundice secondary to biliary stasis. A female in this group was killed in a moribund condition in the final month due to a streptococcal infection of the uterus; all the treated females were in poor condition during the study and failed to gain weight. Urine samples from treated females showed increased numbers of white blood cells which were related to uterine infections. A dose related increase was seen in serum alkaline phosphatase levels in the treated groups, particularly at 75 mg/kg; no changes were seen in serum transaminase levels or any other chemical parameter measured. The weights of testes and pituitary were reduced in all treated males and the treated females showed an increase in uterine weight. Histologically three males and one female at the highest dose showed biliary stasis but no other morphological changes in the liver. The testes and prostate were atrophic in all animals dosed with tamoxifen, treated females showed cessation of ovulation and marked hyperplasia of the germinal epithelium (Fig. 5). This latter change is an exaggeration of the physiological changes occurring in metoestrous. The ovarian effects in females were minimal at 1 mg/kg. The uteri of all females showed severe endometritis with squamous metaplasia; the myometrium had a markedly oedematous connective tissue (Figure 6).

The changes were considered to be related to an *oestrogenic* effect of the compound and this hypothesis was investigated in a further study in which tamoxifen was compared with an oestrogen (stilboestrol). The study was completed in 1966. Four groups each of four female dogs were given daily oral doses for three months. Controls received placebo tablets and the

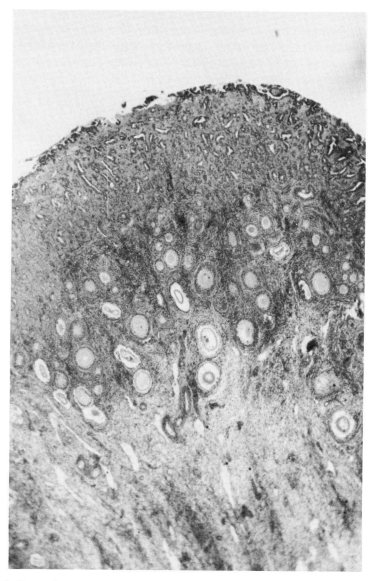

FIG. 5. Ovary from dog treated with tamoxifen showing hyperplasia of germinal epithelium (H&E × 100).

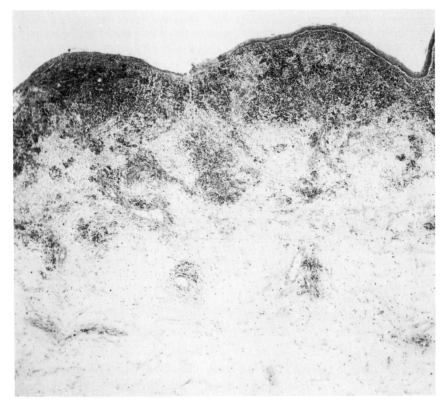

FIG. 6. Uterus from dog treated with tamoxifen showing oedematous myometrium and endometritis (H&E × 100).

treated groups 0.1 mg/kg tamoxifen, 0.1 mg/kg stilboestrol and 2 mg/kg clomiphene respectively. After three months treatment one animal from each group was left undosed for a further month. Blood samples for haematology and clinical chemistry and urine samples were taken at intervals throughout the study. At the end of treatment the animals were killed and necropsied.

Tamoxifen and stilboestrol treated animals showed a marked increase in the uterine weight which was unchanged in the clomiphene group. No significant changes were seen in haematology, clinical chemistry or urine samples. No histological changes were seen in the reproductive tract of the clomiphene-treated animals. The uteri of stilboestrol-treated animals showed an increase in collagen in the myometrium. The tamoxifen treated animals had a diminution in the collagen with fragmentation of the bundles and oedema. After withdrawal of the drugs the uterus returned to normal.

Only the tamoxifen group showed ovarian changes similar to those described in the first study.

The dog uterus is different from the human uterus histologically and in its response to hormones. The endometrium in human and canine species undergoes similar changes when hormonally stimulated. The myometrium of the dog, unlike the human, however, also undergoes considerable change; as oestrous approaches the cells hypertrophy and there is separation and fragmentation of collagen with oedema. The uterine changes seen with tamoxifen did not resemble those produced by stilboestrol or clomiphene. They appeared to resemble an exaggeration of the changes which normally occur in oestrous.

## C. Sub-Human Primates

The pigtail monkey responds to oestrogen by a stimulation of the sexual skin. In ovariectomized animals tamoxifen, at doses up to 20 mg/kg/day, failed to stimulate this swelling, but a dose of 0.2 mg/kg/day antagonized the effective dose of oestradiol. Hence on this tissue in this primate tamoxifen appears to act as a pure antagonist.

To support extended clinical use of tamoxifen a toxicological study in a sub-human primate was considered appropriate and in 1977 a six month test with tamoxifen in the marmoset (*Callithrix jacchus*) was completed. Forty marmosets bred and reared at Alderley Park and all mature (more than 12 months old) were used in four groups each of five males and five females; they were dosed by gavage daily for six months at 0, 0.8, 4.0 or 8.0 mg/kg tamoxifen. Additional animals were dosed in parallel for blood coagulation studies. Blood and urine samples were taken at regular intervals, heart rate and electrocardiograms (ECG) were recorded and the eyes examined by ophthalmoscopy. All of the animals were killed at six months and necropsied. No changes were seen in blood and urine samples, in heart rate or in ECG. A slight increase in ovarian weight was seen in the 8.0 mg/kg group. Histologically the only change seen which was attributable to tamoxifen was an increase in the number of follicular cysts in the ovaries of females dosed 8.0 mg/kg. This effect is related to the *anti-oestrogenic* effect of tamoxifen in the primate (Furr *et al.*, 1979).

## D. Mice

In contrast to the rat, tamoxifen acts as a full oestrogen in the mouse vagina. 1.5 mg/kg/day was the dose which produced cornification in 50% of mice and complete cornification could be obtained at higher doses. Doses of up to 3 mg of tamoxifen per animal were unable to prevent the cornification

TABLE 1. Oncogenicity study in mice: mortality at different times

| Time (months) | | Males Dose/mg/kg | | | Females Dose mg/kg | | |
|---|---|---|---|---|---|---|---|
| | | 0 | 5 | 50 | 0 | 5 | 50 |
| | Number | 25 | 25 | 25 | 25 | 25 | 25 |
| 0–6 | | 4 | 6(1) | 0 | 0 | 3 | 4 |
| 7–12 | | 3 | 6 | 3 | 6(1) | 5 | 5(1) |
| 13–15 | | 2 | 2 | 5 | 4(1) | 0 | 4 |
| Survived to end | | 16 | 11 | 17 | 15 | 17 | 12 |

(  ) No necropsy (cannibalized).

TABLE 2. Oncogenicity study: tumour incidence

| Organ | Type of tumour | | Incidence Males Dose/mg/kg | | | Females Dose/mg/kg | | |
|---|---|---|---|---|---|---|---|---|
| | | | 0 | 5 | 50 | 0 | 5 | 50 |
| | | Number | 25 | 25 | 25 | 25 | 25 | 25 |
| Kidney | Adenoma | | 1 | 0 | 0 | 0 | 0 | 0 |
| Liver | Benign hepatoma | | 2 | 1 | 0 | 0 | 0 | 0 |
| | Malignant hepatoma | | 0 | 1 | 0 | 0 | 0 | 0 |
| Lung | Adenoma | | 1 | 1 | 1 | 0 | 1 | 0 |
| Lymph node | Reticulum cell sarcoma | | 0 | 1 | 1 | 2 | 1 | 0 |
| | Angioma | | 0 | 0 | 1 | 0 | 0 | 0 |
| Ovaries | Granulosa cell adenoma | | — | — | — | 0 | 9 | 9 |
| Pituitary | Adenoma | | 0 | 0 | 0 | 0 | 2 | 1 |
| Spleen | Reticulum cell sarcoma | | 0 | 1 | 0 | 1 | 0 | 0 |
| Testes | Interstitial cell tumour | | 0 | 2 | 21 | — | — | — |
| Thymus | Lymphosarcoma | | 0 | 2 | 1 | 2 | 0 | 1 |
| Tongue | Squamous papilloma | | 0 | 0 | 1 | 0 | 0 | 0 |
| Uterus | Leiomyosarcoma | | — | — | — | 1 | 0 | 0 |
| Vagina | Leiomyosarcoma | | — | — | — | 0 | 1 | 0 |
| | Fibrosarcoma | | — | — | — | 0 | 0 | 1 |

produced by co-administered oestradiol (Jordan, 1976). The drug was also found to be inactive in suppressing oestradiol stimulated increase in uterine weight and to be able, when administered alone, to produce a maximal response similar to oestradiol. At a dose of 1 mg/kg/day tamoxifen could completely inhibit implantation in mice. The oral $LD_{50}$ in mice is 3000 mg/kg and the intravenous $LD_{50}$ is approximately 62.5 mg/kg.

The first oncogenicity study was completed in 1965 and included three groups, each of 25 male and 25 female mice of the Alderley Park (AP) strain 1. They received 0, 5 or 50 mg/kg tamoxifen by stomach tube daily for three months, thereafter in the diet for 12 months (total of 15 months). The test had been designed as an 18 month study but was terminated at 15 months because many of the treated mice had skeletal abnormalities. All but four of the mice were necropsied and all surviving to 15 months were radiographed.

Mortality in each group is shown in Table 1 and indicates that there was no significant difference in mortality in control and treated animals. The incidence of tumours is given in Table 2 and shows that the tamoxifen-treated mice showed an increase in interstitial cell tumours of the testes, more marked at the higher dose, and a similar increase in granulosa cell tumours of the ovary in both treated groups. The majority of tumours were bilateral and all were benign. Gonads and accessory sex organs of treated animals were atrophic and treated females showed cystic endometrial hyperplasia in the uterus (Fig. 7). Minor changes, consisting of fatty change and swelling of parenchymal cells, were seen in the liver of tamoxifen-treated animals. After six months treatment the mice in both treated groups developed a spinal deformity with kyphosis (Fig. 8) due to elongation of the vertebrae and there was a marked increase in the density of long bones and skull (Fig. 9). Histologically the bones showed resorption and new bone formation in irregular patterns (Fig. 10). It was considered that the tumours of the gonads and the skeletal changes were related to an oestrogenic effect of tamoxifen in the mouse. It was known that oestrogens produce interstitial cell tumours in the testes of mice (Hooker, 1948; Gardner et al., 1959; Huseby, 1965) and it was possible that the tumours and the changes were related to oestrogenic activity.

To investigate the hypothesis a second study in mice was designed to compare the effects of tamoxifen with conventional oestrogens. This second study was completed in 1966 and included four groups of AP mice. Since endocrine effects could be influenced by age, each group included ten mice of each sex aged eight weeks at the start (mature), and ten weanling mice of each sex (immature). They were dosed by stomach tube for three months then fed the compounds in the diet for 10 months. The doses used were as follows: 0 Controls, 20 mg/kg tamoxifen, 0.05 mg/kg ethynyloestradiol, 1 mg/kg stilboestrol. Four animals of each sex were killed after three months

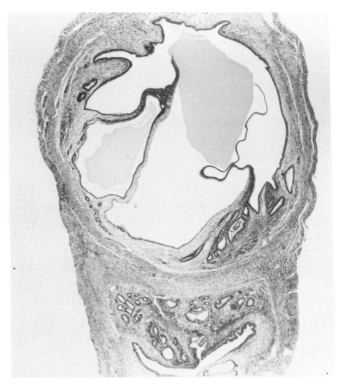

FIG. 7. Uterus from mouse treated with tamoxifen showing cystic hyperplasia of
endometrial glands (H&E × 25).

treatment and necropsied. The remainder were killed at 13 months. Radiographs were taken from one animal of each sex in each group before
treatment and at monthly intervals (in the same animals) for 13 months.

Mortality in all groups was high due to a pulmonary infection with
*Pasteurella pneumotropica*. After 12 months treatment, only 30% of the
animals were still alive and the test was terminated at 13 months. None of the
mice treated with stilboestrol survived to 13 months; the majority had
developed ascites and subcutaneous oedema related to infections of the
urinary tract. No tumours were seen in the mice killed at three months. Mice
dosed with stilboestrol showed cessation of sperm maturation and atrophy
of male accessory sex organs. Mice dosed with tamoxifen showed changes
similar to the first study with cessation of ovulation and cystic hyperplasia of
the uterus. Minor changes were also seen in the liver of all treated mice,
similar to those described in the first study; they were most marked in
animals dosed with ethynyloestradiol. The incidence of tumours, other than

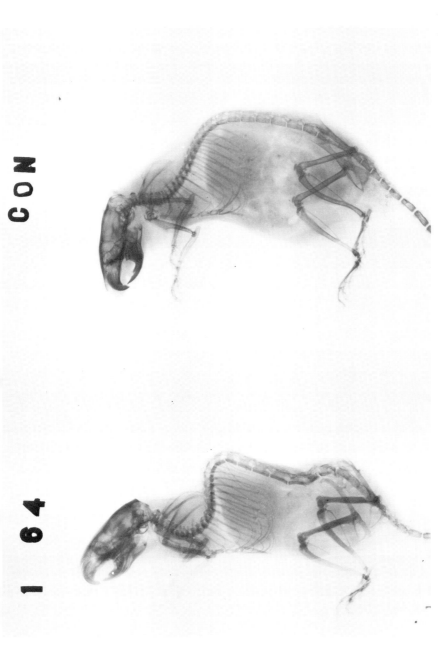

FIG. 8. Prints of radiographs of control (marked CON) and tamoxifen treated mice to show kyphosis in the treated animal.

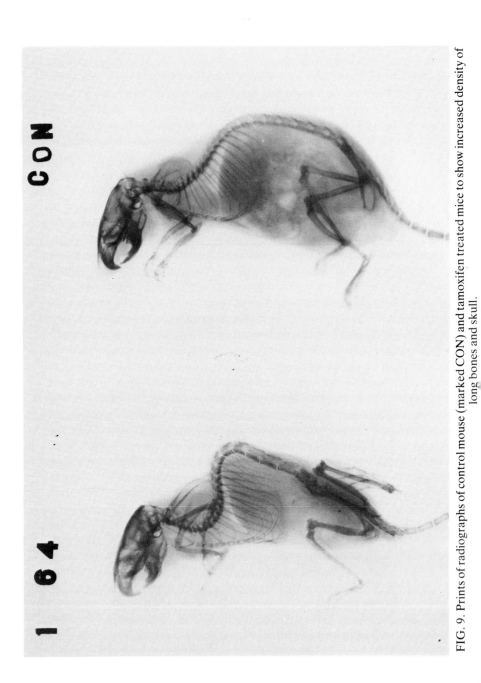

FIG. 9. Prints of radiographs of control mouse (marked CON) and tamoxifen treated mice to show increased density of long bones and skull.

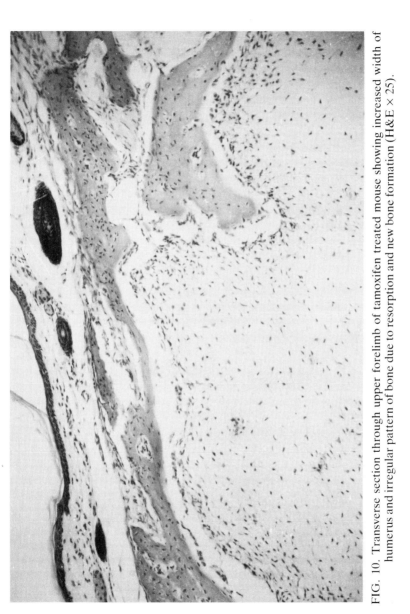

FIG. 10. Transverse section through upper forelimb of tamoxifen treated mouse showing increased width of humerus and irregular pattern of bone due to resorption and new bone formation (H&E × 25).

TABLE 3. Incidence of testicular tumours in mice treated with tamoxifen and conventional oestrogens for 13 months

| Number and age of mice | Control | Tamoxifen | Ethynyloestradiol | Stilboestrol |
|---|---|---|---|---|
| Mature  (10/sex) | 0(0) | 2(0) | 0(0) | 0(2) |
| Immature (10/sex) | 0(0) | 2(2) | 1(0) | 1(0) |

Figures in parentheses indicate the number of mice with hyperplasia of interstitial cells.

those of the gonads, was low and considered to be within the expected spontaneous incidence. The incidence of testicular tumours is shown in Table 3. One female dosed with tamoxifen had a granulosa cell tumour and one female dosed with ethynyloestradiol had a hyperplastic nodule of granulosa cells in the ovary. The smaller number of gonadal tumours in this study, compared with the first, is probably related to the lower dose of tamoxifen and the shorter period of treatment. Since testicular tumours were seen with tamoxifen and the conventional oestrogens and there were none in the controls (and the strain has a very low spontaneous incidence of testicular tumours) it was considered reasonable to conclude that the tumours could be related to the *oestrogenic* activity of tamoxifen in the mouse. Changes in the skeleton consisted of thickening of long bones and skull and elongation of the vertebrae. The incidence of these effects is shown in Table 4. It was concluded that the increased bone density seen with tamoxifen was attributable to its oestrogenic activity. The spinal elongation occurred only with tamoxifen and its aetiology is unknown.

TABLE 4. Incidence of skeletal changes in mice dosed with tamoxifen and conventional oestrogens for 14 months

| Compound | Mice | Thickened long bones and skull | Elongated spinal vertebrae |
|---|---|---|---|
| Controls | Mature | No change | No change |
|  | Immature |  |  |
| Tamoxifen | Mature | ♂ from 6 months | ♂ from 6 months |
|  |  | ♀ from 4 months | ♀ from 5 months |
|  | Immature | ♂ & ♀ from 4 months | ♂ & ♀ from 6 months |
| Ethynyloestradiol | Mature | ♀ from 6 months | No change |
|  |  | ♂ & ♀ from 6 months |  |
| Stilboestrol | Mature | ♀ from 3 months | No change |
|  | Immature | ♂ and ♀ from 3 months |  |

A third study was undertaken in 1967 to examine the effects of tamoxifen at a dose below the median cornifying dose in the mouse. Twenty-five male and 25 female AP mice were fed a diet giving a dose of 0.001 mg/kg/day tamoxifen for 14 months. All of the animals were radiographed and given a full necropsy. No tumours were seen in the gonads and there were no skeletal abnormalities.

## E. Teratogenic Tests

The first study, in the rat, was completed in 1964. Three groups, each of 14 female Alpk/AP rats were pair mated and dosed 0, 0.025 mg/kg tamoxifen from days 1 to 20 of pregnancy, 2 mg/kg tamoxifen from days 8 to 20 of pregnancy. 0.025 mg/kg is the largest dose which could be given throughout pregnancy without completely preventing implantation. At this dose about 50% of matings gave successful pregnancies.

Six rats in each group were killed on day 21 of pregnancy and the foetuses removed and stained with alizarin. The remainder were allowed to raise their young to weaning and the offspring were killed on day 21 post partum and necropsied.

Resorptions were increased and foetal weights decreased in the tamoxifen-treated animals, and three foetuses from two different litters in dams dosed 2 mg/kg showed an irregularity in the ossification of the ribs ("kinky" ribs).

Many additional teratogenic studies were done in the rat to confirm this change; all doses above 2 mg/kg produced an incidence of "kinky" ribs. (Fig. 11). During these experiments it was invariably observed that the uterus of tamoxifen-treated animals appeared unusually tight and it was considered that the *anti-oestrogenic* activity of tamoxifen in the rat might be preventing normal development of the uterus and this was investigated in a further study.

Two groups of 18 female Alpk/AP rats received 0 or 2 mg/kg tamoxifen from days 8 to 21 of pregnancy. On day 21 the dams were killed and various measurements made as follows: the maximum and minimum length of each foetus was measured (still in the uterus and attached to the placenta) by straightening out the foetus and then curling it as much as possible. The difference between the curled and extended length depended on the freedom afforded to the foetus by the uterus, adjacent fluid accumulation and the placenta. The foetuses of control animals were found to have much more freedom of movement than the treated animals. In the tamoxifen-treated animals there was an increase in fluid within the uterine cavity outside the foetal membranes. The histological sections of uterus showed a considerable reduction in size compared with controls.

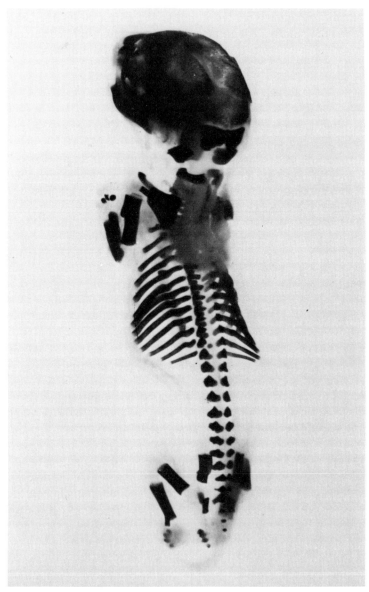

FIG. 11. Print of radiograph of foetal rat from tamoxifen treated dam to show irregular ossification of ribs.

It was concluded that tamoxifen had affected the normal growth of the uterus and that this constriction had affected the growth of the ribs and was not, therefore, a teratogenic effect. This conclusion was supported by the experimental findings which showed that the rib deformity grew out in the early neonatal period, i.e. by day 14 post partum.

A teratogenic test in rabbits at levels of 0.1 and 2 mg/kg tamoxifen throughout pregnancy did not produce any effects on implantation or on the foetus. A study in marmosets at doses up to 10 mg/kg tamoxifen from days 25 to 35 of pregnancy (gestation 138 days) did not produce any effects in the foetus.

## F. Mutagenic Tests

In 1976 tamoxifen was tested in the Ames mutagenic test at levels up to 1 mg/plate; there was no evidence of mutagenic effect under the conditions of this test. A dominant lethal test in rats with tamoxifen at doses up to 9.6 mg/kg for five days did not produce any evidence of a dominant lethal effect.

## G. Pharmacokinetics and Metabolism

Studies using $^{14}$C-tamoxifen in laboratory animals (Fromson et al., 1973) showed that, in rat, mouse, rhesus monkey and dog, the concentrations of total drug-derived material present in plasma were low and that elimination of total radioactivity was slow (Table 5). At that time, despite intensive effort, no satisfactory analytical procedure could be established which would allow measurement of levels of unchanged drug or metabolites in plasma. Hence it was not possible to obtain information on the pharmacokinetics of tamoxifen in laboratory animals without using radioactive materials.

TABLE 5. Pharmacokinetic data in laboratory animals and man[a]

|  | | | | Species | | | | |
|  | Rat | | | Mouse | Monkey | Dog | | Man |
|  | p.o. | i.p. | i.p. | p.o. | p.o. | p.o. | p.o. | p.o. |
|---|---|---|---|---|---|---|---|---|
| Route of administration dose (mg/kg) | 40 | 40 | 1.3 | 40 | 8 | 1 | 5 | 0.3 |
| Maximum serum level ($\mu$g tamoxifen equivalents/ml) | 2.0 | 1.7 | 0.5 | 3.3 | 0.6 | 0.5 | 1.9 | 0.1 |
| "Terminal half-life" (days)[b] | — | — | 10 | 18 | 12 | — | 14 | 9 |

[a] After Froman et al., 1973a. [b] Terminal half-life is derived by assessing linearity of latter portion of the log (excretion rate) versus time plot.

TABLE 6. Routes of excretion of tamoxifen and metabolites in laboratory animals and man.[a]

|  | Rat (i.p.) | Mouse (p.o.) | Species (route) Rhesus monkey (p.o.) | Dog (p.o.) | Man (p.o.)[b] |
|---|---|---|---|---|---|
| % Dose in faeces | 95 | 79 | 65 | 90 | 51 |
| % Dose in urine | 7 | 10 | 19 | 4 | 14 |

[a]After Froman et al., 1973a. [b]Collection at 13 days only.

Equally the systemic levels of radioactivity were insufficiently high to allow the quantitative identification of the component parts. However, it was suggested that the elimination half-life of at least one of the components was long in both animals and man (Fromson, 1973).

Definitive information on tamoxifen pharmacokinetics had to await the (recent) establishment of analytical procedures (Mendenhall et al., 1978; Gaskell et al., 1978; Adam et al., 1980) which, because of the time at which they were developed, have tended to concentrate on the human situation.

Metabolic transformation and routes of elimination were studied by using $^{14}$C tamoxifen. The results (Table 6) showed that in all species examined, including man, the primary route of elimination was via the faeces. Structural identification of several metabolites from faecal or biliary excretion was possible. These metabolites are shown in Fig. 12. Two of these metabolites were also identified in human samples, although recent work in man, using the new specific procedures, has raised doubts as to the validity of the identification of metabolite B (Adam et al., 1979).

## IV. Clinical experience

The first clinical studies with tamoxifen in infertile women were undertaken by Klopper and Hall (1971). El-Sheikha et al. (1972) found that a dosage of 5 mg b.i.d. was only partially effective in causing the disappearance of cystic glandular hyperplasia in patients with menometrorrhagia. In collaboration with Masson, Klopper was able to confirm some of the drug's anti-oestrogenic properties (Masson and Klopper, 1972). They administered it to amenorrhoeic women and showed that, when administered alone, tamoxifen did not induce withdrawal bleeding whilst it was capable of preventing the withdrawal bleeding associated with a short course of ethynyloestradiol.

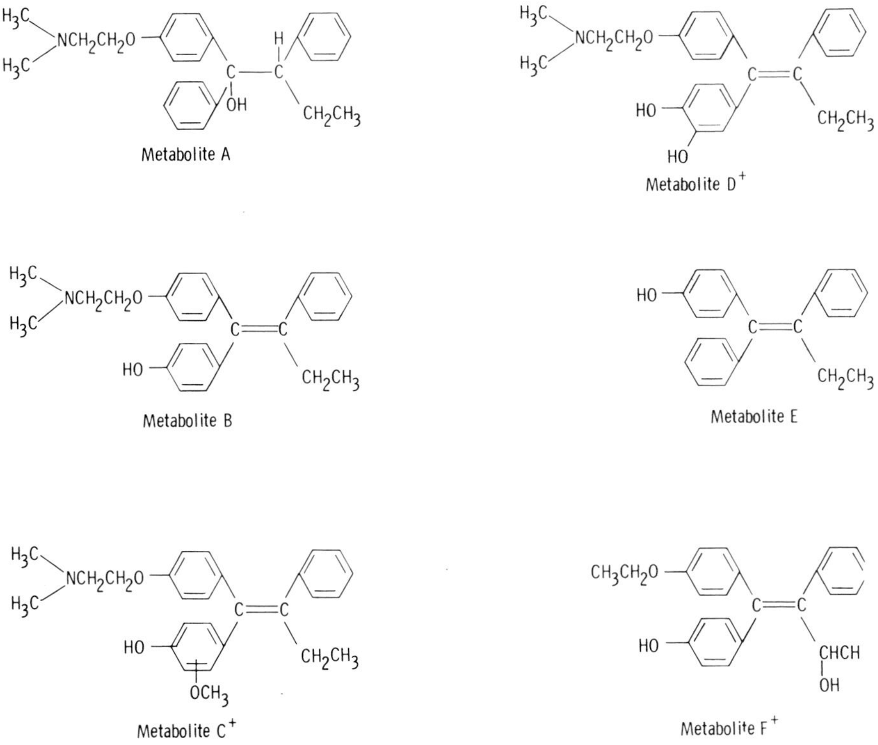

FIG. 12. Structural identification of several metabolites from faecal and biliary excretion.

This early clinical pharmacology suggested that, in the short term, 20 mg of tamoxifen was the minimal consistently effective dose. Some support for this finding has subsequently emerged from studies by Ricciardi and Ian-niruberto (1979) who found that 10 mg tamoxifen per day, given to women with cystic breast disease, did not affect the serum gonadotrophins in normal-cycling premenopausal women. Boyns and Groom (1972), however, found a significant effect (increase in both FSH and LH) in normal-cycling women treated with 20 mg per day. These studies suggest that the threshold for stimulation of pituitary release of gonadotrophins lies between 10 and 20 mg of tamoxifen administered daily.

The situation differs when males are given the drug. Willis et al. (1977) found that 10 mg of tamoxifen per day was capable of producing a consistent rise in gonadotrophins in normal and oligospermic men. The rise was associated with a secondary elevation of both oestrogen and androgen levels. However, they failed to obtain a significant effect upon the sperm count while Comhaire (1976) obtained a significant elevation of the sperm count using 20 mg (2 × 10 mg daily), and this finding has been confirmed by Bartsch and Scheiber (1981). Both Comhaire (1976) and Willis *et al.* (1977) noted that there was no change in the circulating steroid levels in their male subjects. In contrast, Sakai *et al.* (1978) found that female patients with advanced breast cancer develop increases in both sex hormone binding globulin and the cortisol binding globulin following tamoxifen treatment. Thus, it appears that tamoxifen therapy is capable of producing seemingly opposing activities at different target organs and in the two sexes of one species, namely humans.

These early findings of a threshold of consistent activity of tamoxifen which lay between 10 mg and 20 mg daily, led to the institution of clinical trials in advanced breast cancer at the higher dosage. Studies in breast cancer were initiated in 1969 at the Christie Hospital, England. The rationale for the use of an anti-oestrogen was developed from the knowledge that a proportion of breast tumours was oestrogen-dependent. Responses could be achieved by oestrogen withdrawal in both premenopausal and post-menopausal women and by pharmacological doses of oestrogenic agents in postmenopausal women. Even the low circulating levels of oestrogens present after the menopause were felt to be sufficient to stimulate hormone-sensitive tumour growth, and anti-oestrogenic therapy was therefore initiated in post-menopausal women with very advanced disease.

Following the success of the early studies by Cole *et al.* (1971) and Ward (1973), many authors have published papers which cite the use of tamoxifen as a single agent in the treatment of advanced (locally inoperable or recurrent or metastatic) breast cancer in the postmenopausal woman. It is difficult to compare the results of many of these studies because criteria differ for the measurement of response, duration of response and documentation in the studies. Mouridsen *et al.* (1978) have summarized 19 studies from the literature. They noted an overall response rate of 32% (range 16–52%) with a further 21% in the stable disease or "no change" category. The summary by Mouridsen and co-workers was undertaken in an attempt to define the type of patient or tumour which was most sensitive to this anti-oestrogen therapy. While this type of analysis should, ideally, be undertaken in one large study, there were inadequate numbers in some subgroups, even with over 1000 cases in this survey of the literature. A number of interesting points did emerge which are discussed in this section.

## A. The Response in Relation to Other Therapy

Patients previously untreated for advanced disease responded well with a complete and partial response (CR and PR) rate of 118/292 (40%). Prior chemotherapy alone had no effect upon this propensity to respond with 52/112 (42%) of such patients also showing remission. A response to previous endocrine therapy, irrespective of modality, improved the chance of a second remission on tamoxifen to 31/46 (67%). In 34 women who failed to respond to previous endocrine therapy, five (15%) achieved a CR or PR on anti-oestrogen therapy. A small amount of data exists on endocrine responsiveness subsequent to tamoxifen therapy and 7/30 (23%) who failed to respond to this agent subsequently responded to another form of additive endocrine therapy.

Two important points emerge from these data. Firstly, all endocrine therapies cannot be grouped together as "endocrine therapy" with an expected uniform response or failure rate. The assumption that failure to respond to one modality will automatically preclude response to another, is untrue. Secondly response to a first-line endocrine therapy is a better predictor of subsequent hormone sensitivity of the tumour than hormone receptor measurement.

## B. The Response in Relation to Age and Menopausal Status

A surprising feature of the studies is that the response to therapy increases with the age of the patient (Table 7). It is difficult to explain this finding, as one would expect to produce the greatest effects of an anti-oestrogen at a time when oestrogen levels are at their highest, i.e. in younger patients. While this might be a feature of selection of the cases, the fact that free cytoplasmic oestrogen receptor (ER) also increases with age may be a related phenomenon (Spaeren et al., 1973). One mechanistic explanation is as follows. It is thought that the anti-oestrogens act through the free cytoplasmic oestrogen receptor (ER) at the tumour level, and it has been shown, in vitro, that tamoxifen exhibits competitive antagonism of oes-tradiol binding to the ER. As the circulating oestradiol levels fall, with aging, the tamoxifen (which has an affinity for the ER which is considerably lower than the natural ligand) may thus become a more effective competitor and produce greater antitumour effects.

TABLE 7. Response in relation to age of patient[a]

| Age | <50 | 51–60 | 61–70 | >70 |
|---|---|---|---|---|
| CR + PR(%) | 40/126(32) | 58/207(28) | 65/189(34) | 60/126(48) |

[a]After Mouridsen et al. (1978).

The foregoing theory, suggesting a relationship of increasing response with the falling circulating oestradiol levels of aging, becomes untenable when the situation in premenopausal women is examined. Pritchard *et al.* (1979) have published results of an ongoing Phase II study of tamoxifen given to premenopausal women. They have shown a response rate of 11/32 (34%) which, at a dose of 20 mg twice daily and in the face of normal premenopausal oestradiol levels, might not have been predicted if the drug were only competing poorly with postmenopausal oestrogen levels. This study is backed by sporadic reports in the literature of small numbers of premenopausal women who have been treated with tamoxifen. There are 139 such cases published or personally communicated to the author. The response rate of 43/139 (31%) lends support to the finding of Pritchard *et al.* (1979).

Further argument against the theory that the increasing response with aging in postmenopausal women is due to a falling plasma oestradiol level, leading to a better competitive situation for the anti-oestrogens, comes with the findings by Manni and Pearson (1979) and Sherman *et al.* (1979) that circulating oestradiol levels are increased, with a doubling of the ovulatory peak, during continuous tamoxifen therapy. The levels of oestradiol achieved by these women were 30-fold in excess of the normal post-menopausal plasma concentration. This would have been expected to negate or reduce the effect of the anti-oestrogen if simple competition were the only factor involved in its activity—unless the anti-oestrogen were present in a considerable excess. If this excess were present at normal dosages, no increasing response with aging would be expected in post-menopausal women, as tamoxifen to oestrogen concentrations at the cellular level would be well above the top of the dose response curve.

Neither simple competition between oestradiol and tamoxifen nor a large excess of circulating anti-oestrogen can be invoked to explain both the premenopausal and postmenopausal findings described here. Other factors, such as nonspecific protein binding of the two ligands or cell membrane effects of the anti-oestrogen or more subtle changes in the endocrine milieu of the patient, may be responsible for these findings. The most simple explanation, of a change of tumour sensitivity, might also be considered.

## C. The Response in Relation to Dosage

The factors leading to the selection of 20 mg daily as the initial dosage have been discussed above. Ward (1973, 1976) has suggested that 40 mg daily is an optimal dosage, and most subsequent studies have adopted therapy within the 20–40 mg daily dose range.

Table 8 suggests an increase in the response rate at dosages above 20 mg

TABLE 8. Response to tamoxifen related to dosage[a]

| Daily dosage | Patients showing complete or partial response (CR + PR) | Total number of patients treated | Response rate % |
|---|---|---|---|
| 20 mg | 132 | 471 | 28 |
| 30 mg | 34 | 75 | 45 |
| 40 mg | 170 | 432 | 39 |
| 30 mg/m$^2$ | 19 | 44 | 43 |
| 80 mg (37) | 7 | 17 | 41 |

[a] After Mouridsen et al. (1978).

but these data are a summation of results from essentially non-comparable studies. No good dose–response study has been published although two authors, Westerberg et al. (1976) and Elleman (1978, personal communication), have increased the dosage in a number of non-responders, with little improvement. The recent pharmacokinetics data on this drug show a long serum elimination half-life, with a consequently wide scatter in steady state serum levels in patients receiving the same dosage. Coupled with the long time taken to achieve a response in some cases (mean of 70 days to achieve PR in responders) meaningful correlations between dosage and response rate require both the long-term observation of the patient and the measurement of steady state serum tamoxifen concentrations. As the proportion of patients responding to the therapy has been surprisingly similar in all studies, considering the many different prognostic variables present, it is clear that large numbers of patients will be required for future dose–response studies to be meaningful.

## D. The Response in Relation to the Hormone Receptor Status

Much has now been published on the correlation of therapeutic response to endocrine therapy and the presence or absence of the cytoplasmic or nuclear oestrogen receptor protein. There has been an increased predictability of a positive response (CR + PR) in receptor-positive tumour bearing patients, from around 33% in unselected patients to 50–60% in patients selected for therapy on the basis of a positive oestrogen receptor estimation. These data seem to hold true, irrespective of the additive or ablative endocrine therapeutic regimen.

Whilst there is considerable work in progress attempting to raise the predictability of a positive assay to 100%, very little work is in progress in the receptor negative area in relation to endocrine therapies. Good responses are usually reported to occur in less than 10% of receptor negative tumours. Many of the patients whose tumours are classified as receptor negative will never receive any endocrine therapy. If the patients who achieve disease stabilization are included in the analysis (the "no change" group), the predictability of a response in receptor positive cases rises to over 60%, but the receptor negative group becomes "less resistant" to endocrine therapy with 15% or sometimes more of the patients achieving some effect upon the disease (Cheix et al., 1978). This lack of a complete correlation between receptor status and endocrine response would seem to be particularly true for the anti-oestrogens (Bishop et al., 1979). While a 10% good response and a further 5% or more disease stabilization would not suggest that these agents are acceptable first line therapies in receptor negative advanced disease, it would seem that they should certainly be considered after the patient has ceased to respond to first line chemotherapeutic agents.

## E. The Response in Relation to Metastatic Site

The first studies by Ward (1973) and his colleagues suggested that tamoxifen was considerably more effective in soft tissue disease than in the treatment of bone lesions. As a consequence, many clinicians selected patients on this basis for their clinical trials. Morgan et al. (1976) subsequently reported that more bone disease responded in his series than soft tissue disease. Although he is the only worker to find an increase of bone response over soft tissue response, other workers have confirmed that an anti-oestrogen may be effective in these lesions. Mouridsen et al. (1979) showed that soft tissue lesions responded in 35% of cases while 29% of visceral and 25% of bone lesions also responded. Data from a small study by Westerberg (1980) from the Karolinska Hospital, Stockholm, have recently been presented. This comparative study was aimed at comparing bone responses between fluoxymesterone and tamoxifen. There was no difference between the androgen and the anti-oestrogen upon bone disease, confirming the fact that these agents are both to be considered as first line therapy in patients with bone dominant disease.

## F. Side Effects

The data presented above suggest that approximately one-third of untreated patients will respond to therapy with an anti-oestrogen. Those who respond best are older women with no prior therapy or a known response to endocrine therapy and a hormone receptor positive tumour. Much of the data is similar to that produced by classical endocrine therapy with pharmacological doses of oestrogen. However, Stewart (1979), in her comparative study, has suggested that there is a significant prolongation of survival in the anti-oestrogen treated group over those who received diethyl-stilboestrol as first line therapy. An added advantage of the anti-oestrogen is that premenopausal women also respond to tamoxifen therapy.

The major advantage of tamoxifen has been its relative lack of severe side-effects. At normal dosages, less than 3% of patients are withdrawn from therapy due to intolerance. The commonest cause for withdrawal of the therapy is nausea and vomiting. (Hot flushes are probably the most common problem but these do not usually warrant drug withdrawal.) Side effects are very rarely life-threatening and the lack of the common problems associated with oestrogens and androgens has led to the widespread acceptance of tamoxifen.

Recent attention has focused upon hypercalcaemia during therapy. This did not seem to be a common problem in earlier studies but has recently been reported to occur occasionally in the first few weeks of therapy in patients with bony disease (Veldhuis, 1978; Patterson et al., 1978; Spooner and Evans, 1979; Vallalon et al., 1979). The changing pattern of usage of this drug with increasing usage in patients with osteolytic disease, may account for the recent number of reports on the subject. It is difficult to assess the incidence of early hypercalcaemia attributable to the drug, in view of the incidence of spontaneous hypercalcaemia in the disease, especially when there is rapid tumour progression. Drug induced hypercalcaemia would not seem to be a common problem in view of the numbers of patients on therapy in over 70 countries and the relatively small numbers of reported problems. Some workers (Arnold et al., 1979) have attributed the hypercalcaemia to a transient disease flare which often predicted a clinical response.

No cases of acute overdosage of tamoxifen have been described. One study by Kaiser-Kupfer and Lippman (1978) reported upon four women who received between 120 and 160 mg twice daily for periods in excess of 17 months. Retinal and corneal damage resulted in these cases. Perhaps more remarkable is the fact that the drug was otherwise well tolerated for this length of time by all four patients, one of whom had a serum anti-oestrogen level (tamoxifen + N-desmethyl-tamoxifen) in excess of 1500 ng/ml.

## G. Combination Therapy in Advanced Breast Cancer

Following the establishment of tamoxifen as an effective single agent in advanced breast cancer, a number of investigators have assessed the possibility of the drug being integrated into either a combined endocrine approach or in combination with one or more cytotoxic agents.

## 1. Combined Endocrine Therapy

The combinations of cytotoxic agents which act through different cellular mechanisms has revolutionized the approach to the chemotherapy of breast cancer. Little work has taken place with combination of hormonal agents. Many authors have expressed the view that only a fixed one-third of breast tumours are responsive to endocrine therapy—irrespective of the modality employed. The initial experience with combinations employing anti-oestrogen therapy lends some support to this hypothesis (Mouridsen et al., 1979; Mouridsen and Palshof, 1980). Ward (1977) demonstrated that the addition of a prolactin lowering agent to the anti-oestrogen therapy of patients refractory to tamoxifen resulted in further stabilization of the disease, and 2/45 patients had an objective response. However, Settatree et al. (1978) were unable to confirm this finding in women who had not previously received endocrine therapy for advanced disease. The patients in his study received either tamoxifen alone or tamoxifen plus bromocriptine. No clear differences between the two therapeutic approaches emerged in this small, but well controlled clinical trial.

One study alone suggests that combination of the androgen, fluoxymesterone, with anti-oestrogen therapy may improve the responsiveness of tumours. In this study (Tormey et al., 1976), 18 patients received tamoxifen alone and 20 were given a combination of the two therapies. Overall response rates were 5/18 (28%) and 9/20 (45%) respectively (p > 0.1). This interim analysis of small numbers of patients suggests a trend in favour of the combined therapy but larger numbers of subjects are required for a conclusive study. As the dosages of the anti-oestrogen were varied from 2 to 100 mg/m$^2$ twice daily against a fixed fluoxymesterone dosage and the study was conducted in an open fashion, a positive result in favour of the combined therapy in the final analysis needs independent confirmation.

## 2. Combined Anti-oestrogen and Cytotoxic Chemotherapy

The combined approach of cytotoxic therapy with an endocrine manoeuvre has the same attractions as the combination of different forms of cytotoxic chemotherapy; that is, it introduces another therapeutic modality with different dose limiting toxicity and another possible mechanism through which the tumour cell may be attacked. Early uncontrolled studies in advanced breast cancer (Heuson, 1976; Bosch Jose et al., 1977) demonstrated that there is no antagonism between the two classes of agents; in fact, the high response rates suggested that there might even be an additive effect. These results allayed the fears that the cytostatic effects of endocrine therapy might protect a percentage of the tumour cells from chemotherapy. Furthermore, controlled studies have now been reported confirming the initial impression that cytotoxic chemotherapy could be combined with endocrine therapy (Mouridsen and Palshof, 1970; Tormey *et al.*, 1978; Cocconi *et al.*, 1979). None of the studies is very large, but Mouridsen's (a European Organization for Research and Treatment of Cancer (EORTC) study) is ongoing. Tormey's study is interesting in that all patients received dibromodulcitol plus doxorubicin (Adriamycin) as a second line of chemotherapy, which might account for the relatively low response rate of 36% achieved with these agents alone, a rate which increased to 64% in those who received combined tamoxifen therapy. The low response rate (32%) in the CMF (cyclophosphamide, methotrexate, fluorouracil) group of the study cannot be explained away quite so easily. The increase to 58%, by the addition of tamoxifen, would only serve to bring the regimen into the response range claimed by many studies of combination chemotherapy alone. These rates might be explained by the use of stringent response criteria and we must await the publication of the completed study with larger numbers of patients before making firm conclusions.

One important question must be answered if the combined approach is to be favoured above the common policy of giving endocrine and the cytotoxic chemotherapy in sequence. That question is simply, "Does the patient benefit?". Benefit must be measured in terms of an extension of survival time and the quality of life during that time. It is always assumed that neither therapy is curative. The mean duration of response is in the region of one year for the anti-oestrogen and rather less for the chemotherapy, and it has been shown (Henningsen and Amberger, 1977) that responders to the tamoxifen therapy survive longer than the non-responders. However, long-term responders are very rare and virtually all will die of the disease. A comparison of response rates is inadequate for this exercise as the International Union against Cancer criteria only require the response to be maintained for 4 weeks. Thus one patient may develop a partial response after 8 weeks of therapy on a regimen and be dead within a few weeks, due to a rapid progression, while another patient may have a stabilization of her condition for two years. Ironically, the former patient will be classified as a responder to the therapy while the latter is regarded as a treatment failure—or at best a disease stabilization.

Many studies have been published combining chemotherapy and endocrine therapy. Only one study has attempted to ascertain if the improved response rate of the combined anti-oestrogen and chemotherapy is of benefit. Recent results from this study (Cavalli *et al.*, 1978), undertaken by the Swiss co-operation group (SAKK), suggest that there is no clear advantage on disease progression of tamoxifen plus combination chemotherapy (3 regimens) over tamoxifen alone followed by the same chemotherapies. This comparability of both response and survival suggests that the quality of life for the patient might be enhanced by giving the much less toxic endocrine therapy alone as initial therapy. The reverse of this treatment, chemotherapy followed by endocrine therapy, has yet to be compared with the combined modality approach.

The classical tumour kinetic work of Skipper *et al.* (1965) has led us to endeavour to reduce tumour burden by surgery followed by adjuvant chemotherapy in an attempt to effect a cure. Glick *et al.* (1978) and Morgan *et al.* (1976) have both attempted to evaluate the effects of starting cytotoxic chemotherapy during endocrine response when tumour burden is low. They treated initially with the anti-oestrogen alone to reduce the tumour load, and then randomly assigned the patients achieving response or stable disease to receive either combination chemotherapy in addition to the anti-oestrogen or to continue with the tamoxifen alone. The preliminary results of this so-called stage IV adjuvant therapy were encouraging. Glick *et al.* (1980) have recently updated their results. All patients were selected as ER+ or unknown. They were previously untreated and assessment of response was made arbitrarily at 12 weeks on tamoxifen monotherapy. A surprisingly high percentage (71%) of the 89 evaluable patients showed CR, PR or NC considering that the ER status of 40 was unknown. No differences in survival, response or its duration, emerged between the groups randomized to continue tamoxifen plus chemotherapy and tamoxifen alone showed an improvement of their response category after 12 weeks, demonstrating that responses can appear very late with this drug.

It can be seen from publications cited that there is considerable interest in obtaining the answer to the question "How may a safe, effective anti-oestrogen be incorporated into the overall treatment policy, to the best advantage of the patient with advanced breast cancer?". Some of the answers have been found or will be forthcoming but many further studies will be required to delineate the place of tamoxifen in the overall treatment policy.

# H. The Treatment of Male Breast Cancer

The incidence of cancer of the male breast is said to be approximately 1% of all cases of breast cancer. This relatively uncommon tumour would appear to be sensitive to endocrine therapy with responses to orchidectomy occurring in 45–68% of cases (Treves, 1959; Holleb *et al.*, 1968). Ribeiro (1977), in a retrospective review of 200 cases, reported that 38% of patients had responded to diethylstilboestrol with a median remission of seven years. He saw no remission in those who had bone metastases.

Small numbers of patients have received tamoxifen therapy for advanced disease. We have recently reviewed the evidence (Patterson *et al.*, 1980) on data emanating from 16 different centres; 15/31 evaluable cases were classified as responders (CR + PR) and a further five had a stabilization of their disease. Responses were seen in visceral, bone and soft tissue dominant disease and the pattern of response was very similar to that seen in the postmenopausal women. Few side effects were seen. Loeber and Mouridsen (personal communications) reported 2 PR and 3 NC in six patients they treated with the agent. The data suggest that an anti-oestrogen is effective in male breast cancer and deserved consideration as a first-line agent in this disease, especially in those men who have ER positive tumours.

## V. Conclusions

Tamoxifen was originally developed as an oral contraceptive agent and its clinical use for cancer therapy began after the preclinical toxicity studies were complete. Consequently the duration of the studies was much longer than they would have been if the compound had been developed only for cancer treatment. In addition the large number of studies performed was due to the different pharmacological effects seen in the reproductive tract of the various species studied and the need to distinguish which effects were due to agonist (oestrogenic) or antagonist (anti-oestrogenic) activity. In toxicological studies it is standard practice to use very high doses to maximize any toxicological effect. This further complicated the interpretation of studies with tamoxifen which may behave as an agonist at high doses and as an antagonist at low doses in some species. Our understanding of the pharmacological effects of tamoxifen come from the toxicological studies and subsequent biological studies. If such data had been available when the preclinical studies were planned the dose levels selected would have been considerably lower and the additional studies done to explain the effects at high dose levels would not have been required. In retrospect it is clear that the marked agonist activity of tamoxifen in the mouse made it an unsuitable species for oncogenicity studies; the problems encountered (gonadal tumours, bone changes) were related to oestrogenic activity and necessitated two further oncogenicity studies to demonstrate this fact. The development of tamoxifen has shown that when evaluating the safety of such compounds it is of critical importance to select animal species and doses which give similar pharmacological effects to those in man.

In man tamoxifen is one of the few novel therapies which have been successfully introduced into cancer therapy in the 1970's and it has been shown to be useful in clinical problems unrelated to cancer, such as female infertility. The versatility of this agent is enhanced by its relative lack of harmful side effects with less than 3% of patients, at normal doses, being withdrawn from therapy due to intolerance. The most common causes for withdrawal are nausea and vomiting. None of the toxicological studies produced any evidence of vomiting even though high doses were used in dogs which we consider to be a predictive species for vomiting in man. The absence of serious side effects in preclinical toxicological studies has been amply supported by the low incidence of serious side effects in man.

# References

Adam, H. K., Douglas, E. J. and Kemp, J. V. (1979). The metabolism of tamoxifen in human. *Biochem. Pharmacol.* **27**, 145–8.
Adam, H. K., Gay, H. A. and Moore, R. H. (1980). Measurement of tamoxifen in serum by thin layer densitometry. *J. Endocrinol.* **80**, 35–40.
Arnold, D. J., Markham, M. J. and Hacker, S. (1979). Tamoxifen flare. *J. Am. Med. Assoc.* **241**, 2506.
Bartsch, G. and Scheiber, K. (1981). Tamoxifen treatment in oligozoospermia. *Eur. Urol.* **7**, 283–287.
Bishop, H. M., Nicholson, R., Blamey, R. W. and Eston, C. W. (1979). Oestrogen receptors in locally advanced breast cancers. *Proc. Br. Assoc. Surg. Oncol.* Abstr. **41**.
Bosch Jose, F. X., Alonso Munoz, M. C., Ojeda Gonzalez, B. and Viladiu Ouemada, P. (1977). Asociacion de tamoxifen y adriamycin en el tratamiento del carcinoma advanzado de mama. (Combination of tamoxifen and adriamycin in the treatment of advanced breast cancer.) *Oncologia* **80**, 111–113.
Boynes, A. R. and Groom, G. V. (1972). Effect of ICI 46,474 on plasma gonadotrophin concentrations. *In* "Proceedings of a Workshop, ICI 46,474.—Work in progress", pp 35–41. ICI Ltd., Pharmaceuticals Division, Macclesfield, U.K.
Cavalli, F., Alberto, P., Jungi, F., and Mantz, G. (1978). Hormono-chemotherapy versus hormonotherapy followed by chemotherapy in disseminated breast carcinoma. *Med. Oncol.* **5**, Abstr. 17.
Cheix, F., Pemmatau, E., Clavel, M., Mayer, M. and Saez, S. (1978). Cancer évolué dusein: corrélations entre la presence de recepteurs d'estradiol: et la réponse à un antioestrgéne, le tamoxifène. *Nouvelle Press Med.* **7**. 3633–3635.
Clark, E., Dix, C., Jordan, V., Prestwich, G. and Sexton, S. (1978). A comparison, at the cellular and subcellular levels, of the effects of tamoxifen and oestradiol benzoate on the immature rat uterus. *Br. J. Pharmacol.* **62**, 442–448.
Cocconi, F., De Lisi, V., Boni, C., Amadari, O., Poletti, T., and Bertusi, M. (1979); Chemotherapy (CMF) vs combination of hormonal and chemotherapy (CMF plus tamoxifen) in metastatic breast cancer. *ASCO Abstracts* **20**, C-45.
Comhaire, F. (1976); Treatment of oligospermia with tamoxifen. *Int. J. Fert. l.* **21**, 232–238.
Cole, M. P., Jones, C. T. A., and Todd, I. D. H. (1971); A new antioestrogenic agent in late breast cancer: an early clinical appraisal of ICI 46,474. *Br. J. Cancer.* **25**, 270–275.
El-Sheikha, Z., Klopper, A., and Beck, J. S. (1972). Treatment of metrorrhagia with an antioestrogen. *Clin. Endocrinol.* **1**, 275–282.
Eneroth, G., Forsberg, V., and Grant, C. A. (1971). Hydramnios and congenital

cataracts induced in rats by clomiphene. *Proc. Eur. Soc. Study Drug Tox.* **12**, 299–306.

Fromson, J. M., Pearson, S., and Bramah, S. (1973). The metabolism of tamoxifen (ICI 46,474) II In female patients. *Xenobiotica* **3**, 693–5.

Furr, B. J. A., Patterson, J. S., Richardson, D. N., Slater, S. R., and Wakeling, A. E. (1979). Tamoxifen. *In:* "Pharmacological and Biochemical Properties of Drug Substances" (M. E. Goldberg, ed.), Vol. II, pp. 355–399, American Pharmacological Association, Washington.

Gardner, W. U., Pfeiffer, C. A., and Trentin, J. J. (1959). Interstitial cell tumours of the testis. *In:* "Physiopathology of Cancer", 3rd Edition (Ed. F. Homburger), pp. 152–237. Cassell and Co. London.

Gaskell, S. J., Daniel, C. P., Nicholson, R. I. (1978). Determination of tamoxifen in rat plasma by gas chromatography—mass spectrometry. *J. Endocrinol.* **78**, 29–34.

Glick, J. H., Creech, R. H., Holroyde, C., Karpf, M., Torri, S., and Varano, M. (1978). Tamoxifen (TAM) plus CMF for metastatic breast cancer. *ASCO Abstracts* **19**, C-191.

Glick, J. H., Creech, R. H., Torri, S., Holroyde, C., Brodovsky, H., Catalano, R. B., and Varano, M. (1980). *Cancer* **45**, 735–741.

Guiliani, J., Pescatore, D., Gilbert, C., and Martorana, G. (1978). Usefulness and limitation of estrogen receptor protein (ERP) assay in human renal cell carcinomas. *Eur. J. Urol.* **4**, 342–347.

Harper, M. J. K. and Walpole, A. L. (1967). A new derivative of triphenylethylene: effect on implantation and mode of action in rats. *J. Reprod. Fert.* **13**, 101–119.

Henningsen, B., and Amberber, H. (1977). Antioestrogene therapie des metastasierenden mammakarzinoms vier jahrerfahrung mit tamoxifen. *Deut. Med. Wochenschr.* **102**, 713–716.

Heuson, J. C. (1976). Current review of EORTC clinical trials with tamoxifen. *Cancer Treat. Rep.* **60**, 1463–1466.

Holleb, A. I., Freeman, H. P., and Farrow, J. H. (1968). Cancer of male breast. *N.Y. State J. Med.* **68**, 544–553.

Hooker, C. W. (1948). Biology of interstitial cells of the testis. *Recent Prog. Horm. Res.* **3**: 173.

Huseby, R. A. (1965). Factors influencing absorption of medoxyprogesterone acetate. *In:* "Methods in Hormone Research", Vol. 4 (Ed. R. Dorfman), pp. 123–164. New York Academic Press.

Jordan, V. C. (1976). Antioestrogenic and antitumour properties of tamoxifen in laboratory animals. *Cancer Treat. Rep.* **60**, 1409.

Kaiser-Kupfer, M. I., and Lippman, M. E. (1978). Tamoxifen retinopathy. *Cancer Treat. Rep.* **62**, 315–320.

Kistner, R. W. (1965). Further observations on the effects of chlomiphene citrate in anovulatory females. *Am. J. Obst.* **92**, 380–411.

Klopper, A., and Hall, M. (1971). A new synthetic agent for the induction of ovulation: primary trials in women. *Br. Med. J.* **1**, 152–154.

Ljungkuist, I., Terenius, L. (1972). Attachment reaction of rat uterine lumenal epithelium v. suppression of the attachment reaction of some antifertility agents. *Contraception* **5**, 473.

Manni, A., and Pearson, O. H. (1979). Tamoxifen, hypophysectomy and androgens in the treatment of stage IV breast cancer. *Cancer Treat. Rep.* **63**, 1219.

Masson, G. M., and Klopper, A. (1972). The antioestrogenic effect or ICI 46,474 on the human endometrial lining. *In:* "Proceedings of a Workshop, ICI 46,474—

Work in Progress", pp. 27–34. ICI Ltd., Pharmaceuticals Division, Macclesfield, U.K.

Mendenhall, D. W., Kobayaish, H., Shih, F. J. L., Sternson, L. A., and Fabian, C. (1978). Clinical analysis of tamoxifen, an anti-neoplastic agent, in plasma. *Clin. Chem.* **24**, 1518–20.

Morgan, L. R., Schein, P. S., Wooley, P. V., Hoth, D., MacDonald, J., Lippman, M., Posey, L. E., and Beazley, R. W. (1976). Therapeutic use of tamoxifen in advanced breast cancer: correlation with biochemical parameters. *Cancer Treat. Rep.* **60**, 1437–1443.

Mouridsen, H., Palshof, T., Patterson, J., and Battersby, L. (1978). Tamoxifen in advanced breast cancer. *Cancer Treat. Rev.* **5** (3) 131–141.

Mouridsen, H., Ellemann, K., Mattsson, W., Palshof, T., Daehnfeldt, J. L., and Rose, C. (1979). Therapeutic effect of tamoxifen versus tamoxifen combined with medroxyprogesterone acetate in advanced breast cancer in post menopausal women. *Cancer Treat. Rep.* **63**, 171–175.

Mouridsen, H. T., Palshof, T., Engelman, E., and Sylvester, R. (1980). CMF versus CMF plus tamoxifen in advanced breast cancer in post menopausal women. An EORTC trial. *In:* "Breast Cancer: Experimental and Clinical Aspects" (H. T. Mouridsen and T. Palshof, eds), pp. 119–223. Pergamon Press, Oxford.

Patterson, J. S., Furr, B. J. A., and Battersby, L. A. (1978). Tamoxifen and hypercalcaemia. *Ann. Int. Med.* **89**, 1013.

Patterson, J. S., Battersby, L. A., and Bach, B. K. (1980). Use of tamoxifen in advanced male breast cancer. *Cancer Treat. Rep.* **64**, 801–804.

Pritchard, K. I., Thomson, D. B., Meakin, J. W., Myers, R. E., Sutherland, D. J. A., and Mobbs, B. G. (1979). Tamoxifen, A clinical trial in pre-menopausal women with metastatic carcinoma of the breast. *ASCO Abstracts* **20**, C-60.

Ribeiro, G. G. (1977). Carcinoma of the male breast: a review of 200 cases. *Br. J. Surg.* **64**, 381–383.

Ricciardi, IO., and Ianniruberto, A. (1979). Tamoxifen induced regression of benign breast lesions. *Obstet. Gynaecol.*, **54**, 80–84.

Roche, L. M., Gordon, D. L., Barr, A. B., and Paulson, C. A. (1967). Visual changes associated with clomiphene citrate therapy. *Arch. Ophthal.* **77**, 14–17.

Sakai, F., Chiex, F., Clavel, M., Colan, J., Mayer, M., Pommatau, E., and Saez, S. (1978). Increases in steroid binding globulins induced by tamoxifen in patients with carcinoma of the breast. *J. Endocrinol.* **76**, 219–226.

Settatree, R. S., Butt, W. R., London, D. R., Holmes, M., and Morrison, J. M. (1978). Tamoxifen and Bromocriptine combination in advanced breast cancer. *Proc. 12th Int. Cong. Cancer,* Buenos Aeres **9**, 80.

Sherman, B. M., Chapter, F. K., Crickard, K., and Wycoff, D. (1979). Endocrine consequences of continuous antioestrogen therapy with tamoxifen in pre-menopausal women. *J. Clin. Invest.* **64**, 398–404.

Skipper, H. E., Schabel, F. M. Jr., Wilcox, W. S. (1963). Experimental evaluation of potential anti cancer agents XIV Further studies of certain toxic concepts underlying chemotherapy of leukaemia. *Cancer Chemother. Rep.* **45**, 5–28.

Spaeren, U., Olsnes, S., Brennhoud, I., Efskind, J., Pihl, A. (1973). Estrogen receptors in human breast cancer. *Eur. J. Cancer* **9**, 333–357.

Spooner, D., and Evans, B. D. (1979). Tamoxifen and life threatening hypercalcaemia. *Lancet* **2**, 413–414.

Stewart, H. J. (1979). Edinburgh study on "Nolvadex" (tamoxifen) against oestrogens. *Rev. End. Rel. Cancer Supp.* **3**, 51–56.

Tormey, D. C., Simon, R. H., Lippman, M. C. (1976). Evaluation of tamoxifen dose in advanced breast cancer: a progress report. *Cancer Treat. Rep.* **60**, 1451–1459.

Treves, N. (1959). Gynecomastia: the origins of mammary swelling in the male: an analysis of 406 patients with breast hypertrophy, 525 with testicular tumours and 13 with adrenal neoplasms. *Cancer 11* **(6)**, 1083–1102.

Vallalon, A. H. (1979). Hypercalcaemia after tamoxifen for breast cancer: a sign of tumour response. *Br. Med. J.* **2**, 1329–1330.

Veldhuis, J. D. (1978). Tamoxifen and hypercalcaemia. *Ann. Int. Med.* **88**, 574–575.

Ward, H. W. C. (1973). Antioestrogen therapy for breast cancer. A trial of tamoxifen at two doses. *Br. Med. J.* **1**, 13–14.

Ward, H. W. C. (1976). Clinical experience with anti-hormone therapy. *In:* "The Hormonal Control of Breast Cancer". Proceedings of a Symposium at Alderley Park, Sept. 1975, 53–58. ICI Ltd., Alderley Park, Macclesfield, Cheshire.

Watson, J., Anderson, F. B., Alam, F., O'Grady, G. (1975). Plasma hormones and pituitary luteinizing hormone in the rat during the early stages of pregnancy and after post-coital treatment with tamoxifen (ICI 46,474). *J. Endocrinol.* **65 (1)**, 7–17.

Westerberg, H. (1980). Tamoxifen and fluoxymesterone in advanced breast cancer: a controlled clinical trial. *Cancer. Treat. Rep.* **64**, 117–121.

Westerberg, H., Norden Skjold, B., DeSchryver, A., Notte, R. G. (1976). Antioestrogen therapy of advanced mammary carcinoma. *Acta Radiol. Ther. Phys. Biol.* **15**, 513–518.

Willis, K. J., London, D. R., Bevis, M. A. (1977). Hormonal effects of tamoxifen in oligospermic men. *J. Endocrinol.* **73** (1), 171–178.

# 7

# Conclusions

D. R. LAURENCE, A. E. M. McLEAN and M. WEATHERALL

The problems of predicting toxicity in humans from experiments in animals have been known for a long time and remain unresolved. Indeed, a critical review written thirty years ago (Barnes and Denz, 1954), though more applicable to the use of "chemicals" in food and cosmetics than as medicines, needs little amplification to make it applicable today. The extensive arguments which followed the thalidomide tragedy led to various authoritative pronouncements (e.g. Report, 1964) but otherwise revealed that the problems were unchanged. The case for finding out how drugs cause injury to tissues is still crucial, but it does not appeal to a public, a politician or an administrator, who wants to know only "Is it safe or not?" Bureaucratic guidelines or rules for conducting "tests" of toxicity were developed in the U.S. Food and Drug Administration in 1958–63 (Bein, 1963; Zbinden, 1969). They have been copied or adapted elsewhere and have grown whenever a new tragedy occurred or a new test achieved sufficient standing to be added to the requirements. Barnes (1963) predicted that:

> "Testing procedures outlined by authority whether national or international will either be so vague as to be not worth disseminating or become by necessity more precise. The recommended tests would then be carried out by scores of unthinking technicians who will supply a mass of data eventually to be pushed under official noses. The scientific study of toxicology will atrophy and the hazards from new drugs remain as much of a problem in the future as it is today".

The studies in this book provide some evidence with which to examine this prediction.

The key events in the introduction of the seven drugs discussed here are summarized in Table 1. The case histories in the preceding chapters show the kind of evidence which was required at the time, before the drugs were released for widespread use in humans. Of the seven drugs, one, pronethalol, has been withdrawn because it produced tumours in one strain of mice. It did not have a similar effect in four other animal species or in other strains of mice. Its use in man was brief and limited. Another drug, practolol,

TABLE 1. Time scale of introduction of new drugs

| Drug | Synthesized or Discovered | First Published Clinical Studies | First Marketed |
|------|---------------------------|----------------------------------|----------------|
| Bethanidine | 1960 | Montuschi and Pickens (1962) | 1964 |
| Pronethalol | 1960 | Dornhorst and Robinson (1962) | — |
| Propranolol | 1962 | McNeill (1964) | 1965 |
| Practolol | (by 1967) | Symposium (1971) | 1970 |
| Tamoxifen | 1962 | Klopper and Hall (1971) | 1973 |
| Bromocriptine | 1965 | Lutterbeck et al. (1971) | 1975 |
| Cimetidine | 1972 | Symposium (1977) | 1976 |

had widespread clinical use after extensive studies in animals, and was later withdrawn (from long term treatment) because of unacceptable adverse effects in a small minority of patients. Attempts to reproduce these adverse effects, collectively known as the oculomucocutaneous syndrome, in animals have not succeeded; but if the effects are as rare in other species as in man, the scale of animal studies needed would be far beyond the very large and lengthy range which has already been reached. The effects may even be due to a particular human gene and so not be reproducible in animals. All the other drugs produced effects in animals which caused concern and sometimes put further development in jeopardy. Bethanidine seriously impaired fertility in rats, but the mechanism of the effect could be deduced from the known actions of the drug and from reports of clinical experience. Propranolol caused rats to collapse and dogs to vomit severely. Uterine tumours were observed in rats in long term studies and cleft palates in rabbits after very high doses of bromocriptine. Leydig cell hyperplasia and tumours occurred more frequently after cimetidine than in matched controls. In all these studies, determination to proceed led to additional experiments and in the end bringing the drugs into clinical availability. Was their introduction justified and clinical use made safer by these additional experiments? Was the introduction of valuable drugs unnecessarily delayed? Guidelines for toxicity studies generally recommend that some groups of animals receive doses in excess, if necessary greatly in excess, of therapeutic intention, to ensure that toxic effects are produced. When such effects appear it may be interesting to find out more about them, but their relevance to practical therapeutics is questionable. Do the effects of overdose in animals predict target organs in man, and lead clinicians to be appropriately alert? Patients are more likely to suffer from lack of a new drug than from effects of gross overdosage.

On the positive side, both the industrial pharmaceutical developers and the official regulatory authorities gain much comfort from a battery of tests which show that larger doses given for a longer, or relatively longer, time than is proposed for humans, are innocuous to several species of animal. This point of view is explicit in the chapters on tamoxifen and on bromocriptine. It represents a conventional, if uneconomical, attitude to toxicity testing, which leads to an unending proliferation of such tests. The histories presented here suggest that, in development of any drug, some discouraging findings are almost inevitable, and naturally the more tests that are undertaken the more likely is an adverse finding to arise. There are few clear standards of judgement in deciding the significance of particular findings. Differences in tolerance between species, and between strains within species, differences in metabolism between species and between strains, differences in life span, and in duration of dosage can all be argued to make a given result crucial, or negligible, according with the preferred point of view. In such circumstances the comfort given by decisions based on an extended range of tests is largely an illusion.

On the other hand, there is no way of discrediting any particular test or kind of study, especially if it has sometimes led to correct predictions. As long as social and legal sanctions are applied if a drug turns out to have an adverse effect, while no penalties are imposed for failure to discover new remedies, it is inevitable that tests will proliferate, if only to show that both developers and regulators did all they could to minimize hazards. Regulatory safety tests consist of experiments "which have neither an observation as starting point, nor have been designed to test a scientific hypothesis" (Zbinden, 1982). The experiments are done to conform with rules and with no preconception about their purpose except to see whether anything turns up which perhaps ought to be extrapolated to man (Dayan, 1981). Constant critical review of such tests is therefore necessary, both to see whether the experimental results are reproducible and to judge whether interpretations put on them are reasonable. The massive type of study favoured in many official guidelines is immediately suspect, because the opportunities for overlooked experimental errors are substantial and the chance of reproducing the experiment is, on grounds of cost alone, negligible.

It might be argued that much toxicity testing was unnecessary because the substances tested would be, at best, additions to a range of drugs already so numerous as to confuse the prescriber, and introducing new risks without conferring new benefits (except to those who sell them). These are the so-called "me-too" drugs, but the many obvious examples have not clearly been identified as such until some years of clinical experience has shown their lack of greater merit. Many of the most widely accepted and valued drugs have emerged by stepwise modifications. A policy of "no (potential) me-too drugs" would have left us with, say, sulphanilamide and sulphapyridine as the only sulphonamides, and cortisone and hydrocortisone but no prednisolone or betamethasone or dexamethasone. Also, the problems arising when previously unrecognized toxicity appears are much simplified if a good alternative is available. Pronethalol was withdrawn in 1963 without therapeutic difficulties because propranolol was an acceptable alternative. By the time practolol was a source of concern, a number of substitutes was available for prescription.

One way of assessing the value of toxicity testing to contemporary standards is by historical comparison. Records are not easily found of the information available when new drugs were introduced before 1960. Publications describing the pharmacological properties or first clinical use of such drugs sometimes contain a brief account of toxicological studies, involving for instance dosing a few animals of two or three species for as long as a month (hexamethonium; Paton and Zaimis, 1949), or as many as five groups of ten rats for 12 weeks (cyclizine; Norton et al., 1954). Additional studies may have been undertaken but not published when a manufacturer prepared to market the product. Penicillin was evidently used immediately for life saving purposes, because the quantity originally available was minute (Abrahams et al., 1941). It is interesting to note that much testing was done on cell cultures in vitro as a means of assessing safety swiftly and with a minimum of material. When manufacturing was established in U.S.A., further experiments were not so prolonged as to delay the clinical availability later than 1944. One may wonder whether the present regulatory demands would crumble if a situation were to recur in which such urgency of therapeutic need was unmistakable.

If the continued increase in regulatory requirements since the 1950's has served a useful purpose, alarming incidents should now be less common. Serious incidents are sufficiently rare for a significant change of frequency to be difficult to demonstrate, and besides the rate of introduction of new drugs has declined at least in the U.S.A. (Wardell, 1974; May et al, 1983) and to some extent in the U.K. (Griffin and Diggle, 1981). Also, the rigorous definition of a "serious incident" is almost impossible, as it depends on the nature of the ill effect, the condition for which the drug is used, the reliability of reporting, the number of patients involved, the range of national experiences being included and the rapidity or otherwise with which the "incident" came to an end. Table 2 shows a number of reactions which have been recognized since 1945 and which we judge to be important. For reasons given above, it is almost impossible to provide convincing evidence of a change, or absence of change in the discovery of adverse effects in clinical use. Readers may well wish to draw other instances into consideration. But the general

TABLE 2

| Years of Introduction | Drug | Adverse Reaction | Years of Recognition of Adverse reaction | Reference |
|---|---|---|---|---|
| 1887 | Phenacetin | Nephropathy | 1953–1959 | Larsen and Moller (1959) |
| 1931–1955 | Reserpine | Depression | 1954–1959 | Quetsch et al. (1959) |
| | | Breast Cancer | | Anon (1974) |
| 1935 (Japan) | Clioquinol | Subacute myelo-optic neuropathy | 1965–1969 | Meade (1975) |
| 1939 | Diethyl-stilboestrol | Vaginal carcinoma in daughters | 1970–1971 | Ulfelder (1974) |
| 1941–1944 | Penicillin | Allergy and anaphylaxis | 1945–1953 | Idsoe et al. (1968) |
| 1944–1946 | Streptomycin | Auditory and labyrinthine impairment | 1945–1946 | Report (1946) |
| 1949 | Chloramphenicol | Aplastic anaemia | 1949–1952 | Scott et al. (1959) |
| 1951 | Phenylbutazone | Agranulocytosis | 1952–1953 | Fowler (1967) |
| 1953 | Phenothiazines | Dystonia and akathisia | 1956 | Crane (1968) |
| 1956 | Halothane | Jaundice (repeated use) | 1963–1969 | Trowell et al. (1975) |
| 1958–1959 | Thalidomide | Peripheral neuropathy | 1960–1961 | |
| | | Phocomelia | 1961–1962 | Symposium (1965) |
| 1959 | Triparanol | Cataract | 1961–1962 | Kirby (1967) |
| 1960 | Methysergide | Retroperitoneal fibrosis | 1964–1966 | Graham et al. (1966) |
| 1961 | Sympathomimetic aerosols | Death | 1964–1968 | Inman and Adelstein (1969) |
| 1970 | Practolol | Oculomucocutaneous syndrome | 1972–1974 | Wright (1975) |
| 1980 | Benoxaprofen | Jaundice in elderly | 1982 | Anon (1982) |

"Years of introduction" and "Years of recognition of adverse reaction" have a wide range, temporally and geographically; the dates given are approximations. The references are to reviews in which the history of the events can be sought and do not necessarily reflect discoveries of adverse reactions.

trend does not suggest to us a notable reduction of adverse reactions since preclinical testing on a large scale became mandatory, and confirms Barnes's (1963) prediction that "the hazards from new drugs remain as much of a problem in the future as it is today".

If resources are not to be wasted, it is essential to review the enormous amount of information that has been acquired during the "routine testing" of several hundred new drugs. Critical review of such data is difficult, because most reports are submitted to regulatory authorities in strict confidence, and much trouble is taken by regulators to preserve confidentiality (see e.g. Griffin and Diggle, 1981). Such confidentiality may sometimes be desirable to avoid alerting competitors to a company's cherished innovation. It also diminishes the risk of complex technical data being exploited to the company's disadvantage during litigation. The main purpose of this book is to show that data can be made available for public review. We are particularly grateful to the companies which have permitted and cooperated by providing the contributions to this book and for recognizing the general benefit of publication of toxicological findings, and we hope that others will follow their example.

. The examples given here do not, of course, by themselves establish the value of any particular procedure. Indeed, one of the sadnesses of toxicity testing is that we still do not know whether any benefit is gained, except in carcinogenicity studies, by dosing animals for more than one or perhaps three months continuously. The whole process of regulatory testing is an unsatisfactory substitute for scientific toxicology, and we share the widespread view that expansion of regulations prevents the scientific study of toxicity and reduces protection of the patient. But whatever tests, studies or experiments are done, it is as true now as then that:

> "In the last analysis, it is only clinical trials which can reveal whether an effect observed in animal experiments is also relevant to man, and it is only from extensive clinical use of a new compound that valid conclusions can be drawn as to its safety when employed for a specific therapeutic purpose". (Bein, 1963).

The real problem is not toxicological but sociological, how to prevent "mutual escalation" (Zbinden, 1969) of requirements to achieve the negative, and unrealistic, outcome of perfect safety. At present it seems likely that pursuit of this mirage is doing more harm than good. Some of the evidence is here as a basis for better judgement in future.

# References

Abrahams, E. P., Chain, E., Fletcher, C. M., Florey, H. W., Gardner, A. D., Heatley, N. G. and Jennings, M. A. (1941). Further observations on penicillin. *Lancet* ii, 177–189.

Anon (1974). Rauwolfia derivates and cancer. *Lancet* **ii**, 701–702.

Anon (1982). Benoxaprofen. *Br. med. J.* **285**, 459–460.

Barnes, J. M. (1963). Are official recommendations for the testing of drugs for toxicity dangerous? *Proc. Eur. Soc. Study Drug Tox.* **2**, 57–66.

Barnes, J. M. and Denz, F. A. (1954). Experimental methods used in determining chronic toxicity. A critical review. *Pharmacol. Rev.* **6**, 191–242.

Bein, H. J. (1963). Rational and irrational numbers in toxicology. *Proc. Eur. Soc. Study Drug. Tox.* **2**, 15–26.

Crane, G. E. (1968). Tardive dyskinesia in patients treated with major neuroleptics: a review of the literature. *Am. J. Psychiatr.* **124** suppl., 40–48.

Dayan, A. D. (1981). The troubled toxicologist. *Trends in Pharmacol. Sci.* 2/11, I–V.

Dornhorst, A. C. and Robinson, B. F. (1962). Clinical pharmacology of a beta-blocking agent (nethalide). *Lancet* **2**, 314–316.

Fowler, P. D. (1967). Marrow toxicity of the pyrazoles. *Ann. rheum. Dis.* **26**, 344–345.

Graham, J. R., Subj, H. I., Le Compte, P. R. and Sadowsky, N. L. (1966). Fibrotic disorders associated with methysergide for headache. *New Engl. J. Med.* **274**, 359–368.

Griffin, J. P. and Diggle, G. E. (1981). A survey of products licensed in the United Kingdom from 1971–1981. *Br. J. clin. Pharmacol.* **12**, 453–563.

Idsoe, O., Guthe, T., Willcox, R. R. and deWeck, A. I. (1968). Nature and extent of penicillin side-reactions, with particular reference to fatalities from anaphylactic shock. *Bull. World Heath Org.* **38**, 159–188.

Inman, W. H. W. and Adelstein, A. M. (1969). Rise and fall of asthma mortality in England and Wales in relation to use of pressurized aerosols. *Lancet* **ii**, 279–284.

Kirby, T. J. (1967). Cataracts produced by triparanol. (MER/29) *Trans. Am. Ophth. Soc.* **65**, 493–543.

Klopper, A. and Hall, M. (1971). A new synthetic agent for the induction of ovulation: primary trials in women. *Br. med. J.* **1**, 152–154.

Larsen, K. and Moller, C. E. (1959). A renal lesion caused by abuse of phenacetin. *Acta med. Scand.* **164**, 53–71.

Lutterbeck, P. M., Pryor, S., Varga, L. and Wenner, R. (1971). Treatment of non-puerperal galactorrhoea, with an ergot alkaloid. *Br. med. J.* **3**, 228–229.

McNeil, R. S. (1971). The effects of beta-agonists on the bronchi. *Postgrad. Med. J.* **47** (Suppl.), 14–16.

Meade, T. W. (1975). Subacute myelo-optic neuropathy and clioquinol. An epidemiological case-history for diagnosis. *Br. J. prev. soc. Med.* **29**, 157–169.

Montuschi, E. and Pickens, P. T. (1962). A clinical trial of two related adrenergic neurone blocking agents—BW392C60 and BW467C60. *Lancet* **ii**, 897–901.

Norton, S., Colville, K. I., Light, A. E., Wnuck, A. L., Fanelli, R. V. and de Beer, E. J. (1954). Pharmacologic properties of cyclizine hydrochloride (marezine). *J. Pharmacol. exp. Ther.* **112**, 297–305.

Paton, W. D. M. and Zaimis, E. J. (1949). The pharmacological actions of polymethylene bistrimethylammonium salts. *Br. J. Pharmacol.* **4**, 381–400.

Quetsch, R. M., Achor, R. W. P., Litin, E. M. and Faucett, R. L. (1959). Depressive reactions in hypertensive patients. *Circulation* **19**, 366–375.

Report (1946). Streptomycin in the treatment of infections. A report of one thousand cases. *J. Am. med. Ass.* **132**, 4–11, 70–77.

Report (1964). First report of the expert committee on drug toxicity. London, Association of the British Pharmaceutical Industry.

Scott, J. L., Cartwright, G. E. and Wintrobe, M. M. (1959). Acquired aplastic anaemia: an analysis of thirty-nine cases and review of the pertinent literature. *Medicine (Baltimore)* **38**, 119–172.

Symposium (1965). "Embryopathic Activity of Drugs". London, Churchill.

Symposium (1971). Practolol in the management of cardiac dysrhythmias following myocardial infarction and cardiac surgery. *Postgrad. Med.* **5, 47** (Suppl.), 25–29.

Symposium (1977). "Cimetidine". Amsterdam, Excerpta Medica.

Trowell, J., Peto, R. and Crampton Smith, A. (1975). Controlled trial of repeated halothane anaesthetics in patients with carcinoma of the uterine cervix treated with radium. *Lancet* **i**, 821–823.

Ulfelder, H. (1973). Stilbestrol, adenosis and adenocarcinoma. *Am. J. Obst. Gyn.* **117**, 794–798.

Venning, G. R. (1983). Identification of adverse reactions to new drugs. *Br. med. J.* **286**, 199–202, 289–292, 365–368, 458–460, 544–547.

Wardell, W. M. (1974). Therapeutic implications of the drug lag. *Clin. Pharmacol. Ther.* **15**, 73–96.

Wardell, W. M. (1978). The drug lag revisited: comparison by therapeutic area of patterns of drugs marketed in the United States and Great Britain from 1972 through 1976. *Clin. Pharmacol. Ther.* **24**, 499–594.

Wright, P. (1975). Untoward effects associated with practolol administration: oculomucocutaneous syndrome. *Br. med. J.* **1**, 595–600.

Zbinden, G. (1969). Drug safety: experimental programme. *Science* **164**, 643–647.

Zbinden, G. (1982). Current trends in safety testing and toxicological research. *Naturwissenschaften* **69**, 255–259.

# Index

**Note:** Each chapter contains references to a large number of negative results, seldom involving more than a word or two of text. Such negative results are easily located, and are not cited in this index.